Vertebroplasty and Kyphoplasty

Thieme

Vertebroplasty and Kyphoplasty

Daniel K. Resnick, M.D., M.S.
Associate Professor of Neurosurgery
Department of Neurosurgery
University of Wisconsin
Madison, Wisconsin

Steven R. Garfin, M.D.
Professor and Chair
Department of Orthopedic Surgery
University of California–San Diego
San Diego, California

Thieme
New York • Stuttgart

Thieme Medical Publishers, Inc.
333 Seventh Ave.
New York, NY 10001

Editor: Tim Hiscock
Vice President, Production and Electronic Publishing: Anne T. Vinnicombe
Production Editor: Print Matters, Inc.
Marketing Director: Phyllis Gold
Sales Manager: Ross Lumpkin
Chief Financial Officer: Peter van Woerden
President: Brian D. Scanlan
Compositor: Compset, Inc.
Printer: Maple-Vail Manufacturing Company

Library of Congress Cataloging-in-Publication Data

Vertebroplasty and kyphoplasty / [edited by] Daniel K. Resnick and Steven R. Garfin.
    p. ; cm.
    Includes bibliographical references and index.
    ISBN 1-58890-227-7 (US : HC) — ISBN 3-13-135341-4 (GTV : HC)
       1. Spine—Surgery. 2. Spine—Fractures—Surgery. 3. Osteoporosis—Complications. 4. Orthopedics.
    [DNLM: 1. Spinal Fractures—surgery. 2. Fractures, Spontaneous—surgery. 3. Orthopedic Procedures—
    methods. 4. Osteoporosis—complications. WE 725 V567 2005] I. Resnick, Daniel K. II. Garfin,
    Steven R.
    RD768.V465 2005
    617.5'6059—dc22   2004062056

Important note: Medical knowledge is ever-changing. As new research and clinical experience broaden our knowledge, changes in treatment and drug therapy may be required. The authors and editors of the material herein have consulted sources believed to be reliable in their efforts to provide information that is complete and in accord with the standards accepted at the time of publication. However, in view of the possibility of human error by the authors, editors, or publisher of the work herein or changes in medical knowledge, neither the authors, editors, or publisher, nor any other party who has been involved in the preparation of this work, warrants that the information contained herein is in every respect accurate or complete, and they are not responsible for any errors or omissions or for the results obtained from use of such information. Readers are encouraged to confirm the information contained herein with other sources. For example, readers are advised to check the product information sheet included in the package of each drug they plan to administer to be certain that the information contained in this publication is accurate and that changes have not been made in the recommended dose or in the contraindications for administration. This recommendation is of particular importance in connection with new or infrequently used drugs.

Some of the product names, patents, and registered designs referred to in this book are in fact registered trademarks or proprietary names even though specific reference to this fact is not always made in the text. Therefore, the appearance of a name without designation as proprietary is not to be construed as a representation by the publisher that it is in the public domain.

5 4 3 2 1

TMP ISBN 1-58890-227-7
GTV ISBN 3-13-135341-4

Acknowledgment

The editors would like to thank the contributors to this text for their hard work and patience. Vertebral augmentation procedures are an important part of the spine practitioner's armamentarium. There are several procedures available for vertebral augmentation and several viewpoints regarding the relative benefits of these procedures. We appreciate the professionalism and honesty of our contributors and value the insights that they have shared.

CME Credit Information

The American Association of Neurological Surgeons (AANS) is accredited by the Accreditation Council for Continuing Medical Education to sponsor continuing medical education for physicians.

The American Association of Neurological Surgeons designates this continuing medical education activity for a maximum of 15 credits in Category I of the Physician's Recognition Award of the American Medical Association.

The Home Study Examination is online on the AANS web site at www.aans.org/education/books/vertebro.asp.

Participants have until February 28, 2007 to complete and pass the examination. No CME will be available after this date. For more information on CME credits, visit the AANS web site http://www.aans.org/education/cme.asp or contact the Member Services Department of the AANS at

Phone: (888) 566-AANS (2267) or (847) 378-0500
E-mail: memberservices@aans.org

Contents

Preface

Vertebral compression fractures are a major cause of morbidity in the aging population. These fractures have traditionally been treated with immobilization and pain medications. In the last decade, vertebroplasty and subsequently kyphoplasty have emerged as treatments for these fractures. The use of these techniques has expanded exponentially over the last several years. This phenomenon is largely fueled by the fact that no competing treatment exists that can provide such immediate pain resolution and stability to the osteoporotic spine. The fact that these goals can be accomplished minimizing the extent of incisions in an awake patient make these procedures even more appealing.

There exists substantial controversy among physicians who perform these procedures regarding a number of key issues. For example, there is no agreement as to which procedure is preferable. There are no real guidelines as to when patients with acute fractures should be treated. It is also unclear what role these procedures play in non-osteoporotic pathological compression fractures, burst fractures, or as a supplement to traditional spinal stabilization procedures. The long-term outcome of patients treated with these procedures is only now beginning to be able to be assessed and there are questions as to what effects these procedures have on adjacent level disease. There is very little information available regarding complication management. Finally, there is absolutely no agreement as to what the training requirements should be for practitioners.

The purpose of this text is to explore these issues in a comprehensive, fair, and balanced fashion. The panel of authors includes interventional radiologists, neurosurgeons, and orthopedic surgeons who are well versed in the procedures. By juxtaposing the radiologist's perspective and the surgeon's perspective, we hope to allow the reader to judge for him or herself what the important similarities and differences are between the procedures and the specialists who perform them. In several instances, we have asked experts with different training backgrounds and different practice patterns to comment on similar topics. For example, chapters on techniques and complication avoidance have been prepared by both radiologists and surgeons, allowing a direct comparison by the reader. As any practitioner knows, complications occur. The causes, nature, and ways of addressing of the more common complications are presented in several chapters. We have included a discussion of emerging technologies and a discussion regarding the practicalities of incorporating these procedures into an active spine practice.

As new technologies are introduced into the armamentarium of spine practitioners, it is important to critically evaluate them. Costs, complications, and the effort spent to acquire new skills must be offset by improvements in patient outcomes. This text represents a snapshot of what is known about the ability of vertebroplasty and kyphoplasty to improve patient outcomes. Experienced practitioners also offer tips to lower the incidence of complications. As this rapidly developing field progresses, new information will become available. The reader is encouraged to use this text as a means to understand the basic principles of both procedures and as a reference for comparison to the evolving literature.

Contributors

Raju Balahadra, M.D.
Department of Neurosurgery
Wayne State University
Detroit, Michigan

D. W. Cahill, M.D.†
Department of Neurosurgery
University of South Florida
Tampa, Florida

R. V. Chavali
Assistant Professor
Department of Radiology
Section of Neuroradiology
Boston University School of Medicine
Boston, Massachusetts

I. S. Choi, M.D.
Burlington Interventional Radiology
Lahey Medical Center
Burlington, Massachusetts

Jacques E. Dion, M.D., F.R.C.P.(P.)
Professor of Radiology and Neurosurgery
Department of Radiology
Emory University Hospital
Atlanta, Georgia

Richard D. Fessler, M.D.
Department of Neurosurgery
Wayne State University
Detroit, Michigan

Richard G. Fessler, M.D.
John Harper Seeley Professor and Chief
Section of Neurosurgery
University of Chicago Hospitals
Chicago, Illinois

Steven R. Garfin, M.D.
Professor and Chair
Department of Orthopedic Surgery
University of California–San Diego
San Diego, California

Peter C. Gerszten, M.D., M.P.H.
Assistant Professor
Department of Neurological Surgery and
    Radiation Oncology
Presbyterian University Hospital
Pittsburgh, Pennsylvania

Jeffrey D. Gross, M.D.
Medical Director
Orthopedic and Spine Injury Specialists
Laguna Niguel, California

---

†Deceased

Lisa L. Guyot, M.D., Ph.D.
Department of Neurosurgery
Wayne State University
Detroit, Michigan

James S. Harrop, M.D.
Assistant Professor
Department of Neurosurgery
Thomas Jefferson University
Philadelphia, Pennsylvania

Robert Q. Ingraham, M.D.
Division of Neurosurgery
University of Tennessee Graduate School of Medicine
Knoxville, Tennessee

Toru Koizumi, M.D.
Department of Neurosurgery
Saga Medical School
Saga, Japan

Isador Lieberman, M.D., M.B.A., F.C.S.(C.)
Professor of Surgery
Director, Minimally Invasive Surgery Center
Cleveland Clinic Spine Institute
Cleveland, Ohio

John M. Mathis, M.D.
Chairman
Department of Radiology
Lewis-Gale Medical Center
Salem, Virginia

Geoffrey McCullen, M.D.
Orthopedic Spine Surgery
Neurological and Spinal Surgery, LLC
Lincoln, Nebraska

D. M. Melton, M.D.
Department of Neurosurgery
University of South Florida
Tampa, Florida

Roham Moftakhar, M.D.
Department of Neurosurgery
University of Wisconsin School of Medicine
Madison, Wisconsin

T. Glenn Pait, M.D.
Department of Neurosurgery
University of Arkansas
Little Rock, Arkansas

Mick J. Perez-Cruet, M.D., M.S.
Director, Minimally Invasive Spinal Surgery
Rush-Presbyterian St. Luke's Medical Center
Chicago, Illinois
Associate Director, Institute for Spine Care
Silver Cross Hospital
Joliet, Illinois

Frank M. Phillips, M.D.
Professor,
Department of Orthopedic Surgery
Rush University Medical Center
Chicago, Illinois

Mark A. Reiley, M.D.
Berkeley Orthopedic Group
Berkeley, California

Daniel K. Resnick, M.D., M.S.
Associate Professor of Neurosurgery
Department of Neurosurgery
University of Wisconsin
Madison, Wisconsin

Marcelo A. Rodrigues
Department of Orthopedics
University of California–San Francisco
University Medical Center
Fresno, California

H. Claude Sagi, M.D.
Florida Orthopedic Institute
Orthopedic Trauma Service
Tampa General Hospital
Tampa, Florida

Faheem A. Sandhu, M.D., Ph.D.
Assistant Professor
Department of Neurosurgery
Georgetown University Hospital
Washington

J. S. Sarzier, M.D.
Department of Radiology and Neurosurgery
Division of Neurointerventional Radiology
University of South Florida
Tampa, Florida

Byron Gregory Thompson, M.D.
Department of Neurosurgery
University of Michigan Medical Center
Ann Arbor, Michigan

Frank C. Tong, M.D.
Assistant Professor of Radiology and Neurosurgery
Department of Radiology
Emory University Hospital
Atlanta, Georgia

Eeric Truumees, M.D.
Attending Surgeon
Section of Spinal Surgery
Department of Orthopedic Surgery
Orthopaedic Director
Gehring Biomechanic Laboratory
William Beaumont Hospital
Royal Oak, Michigan

William C. Welch, M.D., FACS
Chief and Associate Professor
Department of Neurological Surgery
Presbyterian University Hospital
Pittsburgh, Pennsylvania

Brian P. Witwer, M.D.
Chief Resident
Department of Neurosurgery
University of Wisconsin
Madison, Wisconsin

Wade H. Wong, M.D.
Professor of Radiology
University of California–San Diego
Thornton Hospital
La Jolla, California

Hansen A. Yuan, M.D.
Professor
Department of Orthopedic and Neurological
    Surgery
State University of New York
Upstate Medical University
Syracuse, New York

Vertebroplasty and Kyphoplasty

1

Vertebroplasty and Kyphoplasty: An Overview

FAHEEM A. SANDHU, BYRON GREGORY THOMPSON, MICK J. PEREZ-CRUET, AND RICHARD G. FESSLER

Objectives: On completion of this chapter, the reader should be able to (1) list the most common sequelae of vertebral compression fractures in the elderly and (2) summarize currently available treatment options.

Accreditation: The American Association of Neurological Surgeons is accredited by the Accreditation Council for Continuing Medical Education to sponsor continuing medical education for physicians.

Credit: The American Association of Neurological Surgeons designates this continuing medical education activity for a maximum of 15 credits in Category I of the Physician's Recognition Award of the American Medical Association.

The Home Study Examination is online at www.aans.org/education/books/vertebro.asp

Spinal compression fractures, most commonly caused by osteoporosis, are a significant cause of morbidity and mortality in the elderly population.[1] Almost one fourth of women over the age of 50 are afflicted by osteoporotic bone fractures.[2] Risk of developing compression fractures increases with age; in women 80 to 85 years of age, up to 40% suffer osteoporotic bone fractures.[3] Additional risk factors for developing osteoporotic compression fractures include menopause, chronic steroid therapy, prolonged immobilization, and renal insufficiency. Estimates of the cost of osteoporotic bone fractures in 1995 approached $750 million in the United States alone.[4]

Osteoporosis, a systemic disease, is the most common metabolic bone disorder, affecting greater than 24 million Americans.[4] Progressive loss of bone matrix and mineralization occur, leaving the vertebral column vulnerable to the development of compression fractures after minimal to no trauma.[5] The pain caused by vertebral fractures may last months and prove to be severely debilitating. Unfortunately, the use of primarily medical therapy occasionally results in narcotic dependence. In a predominantly elderly population, this can alter mood and mental status, thus compounding the patient's condition.[6] Chronic pain, sleep loss, depression, decreased

mobility, and loss of independence are all sequelae of vertebral compression fractures.[7,8] Additionally, both thoracic and lumbar compression fractures decrease lung capacity.[9]

Conservative treatment begins with sufficient pain medication and bed rest. Physical therapy and bracing are added and by 4 to 6 weeks, pain usually subsides. The majority of vertebral compression fractures that come to clinical attention are treated conservatively. However, bed rest accelerates bone loss and increases the risk of developing deep venous thromboses, which negatively impacts the patient.[10,11] Additionally, muscles become deconditioned, which, in combination with bone loss, may exacerbate pain symptoms and decrease independence; therefore, an argument can rationally be made to treat vertebral compression fractures much more aggressively.

Percutaneous vertebroplasty and kyphoplasty are recent developments in the treatment of compression fractures. The goal of vertebroplasty is conferring strength and stability to a vertebra. Kyphoplasty attempts to restore vertebral body height in addition to increasing strength. Currently, both are used in the treatment of osteoporotic as well as steroid-induced compression fractures, spine metastases, and vertebral

1

hemangiomas.[12–15] Vertebroplasty and kyphoplasty are effective in strengthening both normal and osteoporotic cadaveric bone. Several different bone cements used in these procedures have been found to restore the vertebral body strength to normal or even greater than normal.[16] Both bilateral and unilateral injections of bone cement have been found to increase the strength of osteoporotic cadaveric bone.[17] This chapter summarizes the indications, techniques, and complications of both vertebroplasty and kyphoplasty procedures.

■ Indications for Vertebroplasty

Ideal candidates for vertebroplasty are patients who have failed conservative therapy and continue to have pain that negatively affects mobility and activities of daily living. Pain should be localizable to the fracture level. We select patients whose duration of pain from fracture is greater than 6 weeks but less than 1 year. Others have successfully treated painful fractures of 2 years' duration.[12] Contraindications for vertebroplasty include severe wedge deformity with loss of greater than 90% of vertebral height (vertebra plana), comminuted burst fracture, spinal canal compromise >20%, epidural tumor extension, inability to lie prone, uncorrected coagulopathy, and inability to localize the source of pain. Vertebroplasty should be done only when the ability to perform emergent decompression surgery is readily available. Use of computed tomography (CT) guidance may improve safety in this situation. Vertebroplasty may also be used in the treatment of destructive vertebral body hemangiomas and metastases. Disruption of the posterior cortex of the vertebral body is a relative, but not an absolute, contraindication for performing vertebroplasty. However, extra care must be taken to ensure that extravasation of bone cement into the spinal canal does not occur.

■ Preoperative Evaluation

Prior to the procedure, it is necessary to perform a complete neurologic examination documenting any motor or sensory anomalies in addition to identifying any existing radiculopathies. The preprocedural evaluation, at a minimum, should include anteroposterior (AP) and lateral radiographs of the spine; a CT is performed to evaluate the posterior cortex for any disruptions that may increase the risk of cement leakage into the spinal canal during the procedure and to determine if there is any extension of pathology into the spinal canal. Localization of the symptomatic level may prove difficult and acquisition of a bone scan in

these individuals is often helpful. Magnetic resonance imaging (MRI), though not mandatory, is strongly recommended.

■ Vertebroplasty Procedure

Vertebroplasty is a procedure whereby bone cement is introduced into a fractured vertebral body via a minimally invasive, percutaneous injection. It was developed with the goals of decreasing pain from symptomatic compression fractures, strengthening the spine, and improving mobility.[18,19] Stabilization of bone may be effective in preventing the progression of kyphosis and shortening the duration of pain. An 11-gauge needle is usually used for the delivery of polymethylmethacrylate (PMMA) (Codman cranioplast type 1; CMN Laboratories, Blackpool, England) into the fractured vertebra via a transpedicular route.

The procedure may be performed in the operating room, but an angiographic suite that is equipped with fluoroscopy and basic surgical supplies is recommended (Fig. 1–1). Once venous access is obtained, an anesthetist can administer sedatives and analgesics; it is ideal to have an awake and interactive patient. Oxygen saturation, blood pressure, and heart rate are closely monitored during the procedure. The patient is situated in the prone position on a Wilson frame or chest rolls. The patient's arms are placed above the shoulders, joints are slightly flexed, and adequate padding is placed beneath potential pressure points. The thoracic and lumbar spine must remain free of radiopaque objects when using fluoroscopy.

Adherence to strict sterile protocol is the standard of practice throughout the procedure. Patients undergoing this procedure may have significant osteopenia and marked kyphotic and scoliotic changes that make localization of the appropriate level difficult. A radiopaque marker can be utilized to aid localization of the appropriate level; both lateral and AP projections are used to visualize the pedicle of the vertebral body to be treated. Once identified, a mark is placed on the skin overlying the pedicle of interest. Following administration of lidocaine (Abbot Laboratories; Chicago, IL) at the skin entry site, a 21-gauge spinal needle is inserted and docked onto the pedicle in question. Lateral fluoroscopy is used to verify the correct trajectory. Then lidocaine with epinephrine (Abbot Laboratories) is injected into the soft tissue and the periosteum. A scalpel is used to create a stab incision, lateral to the midline at the point previously marked to identify the pedicle, through which an 11-gauge bone biopsy needle is introduced. The biopsy needle is guided along the same path as the spinal needle and docked onto the medial third of the pedicle. AP fluoroscopy is used to confirm trajectory. Using the

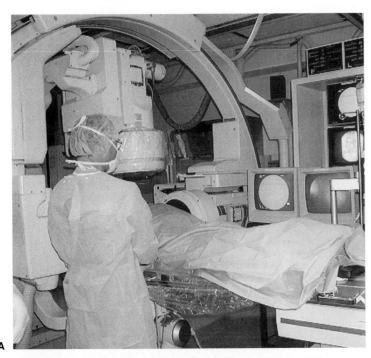

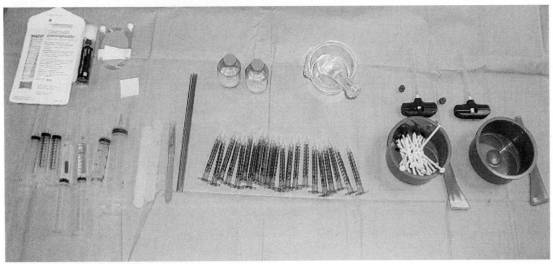

FIGURE 1–1 (A) Patient positioning and angiography suite setup with biplanar fluoroscopy. **(B)** Basic surgical supplies needed to perform percutaneous vertebroplasty.

A

B

"bull's eye" technique, the biopsy needle is then embedded ~5 to 10 mm into the pedicle. The entire length of the needle image should be located within the pedicle. This is potentially the most painful part of the procedure, and administration of sedatives and analgesics immediately prior to needle insertion into the pedicle is prudent.

When insertion of the biopsy needle is complete, lateral fluoroscopic views are acquired. The lateral view ensures that the biopsy needle is appropriately directed along the axis of the pedicle, whereas the AP view confirms that the tip of the needle is in the medial third of the pedicle. Using lateral fluoroscopy, the needle is manually advanced with a slow, twisting motion until the tip is in the anterior one third of the vertebral body

(Fig. 1–2). At this point, the AP view should demonstrate the needle tip as being in the midbody.

To avoid introduction of air during the injections, the needle is filled with sterile saline following adequate placement. Accurate placement of the needle in the anterior third of the vertebral body is necessary because the anterior half of the vertebral body sustains 80% of the load that the anterior column supports. Moreover, the main venous drainage of the vertebral body begins at the midpoint of the anterior–posterior dimension of the vertebral body. Violation of the pedicle cortex should be avoided because it can lead to extrusion of PMMA into the neural foramen and subsequent radiculopathy.

Contrast dye, delivered via a 10-cc syringe with a short piece of pressure tubing, is used to visualize vertebral

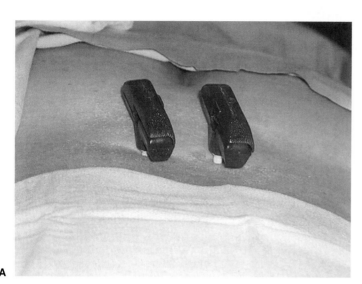
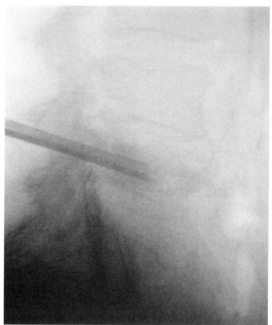

A   B

FIGURE 1–2 (A) Percutaneous access to both pedicles with 11-gauge biopsy needles. **(B)** Radiographic confirmation of adequate placement of the needles is obtained on lateral fluoroscopy.

venous drainage under continuous fluoroscopy. Typically, the contrast should slowly accumulate within the vertebral body and then drain via segmental veins (Fig. 1–3). Digital subtraction angiography aids in the visualization of the injection and runoff. If the contrast runoff from the vertebra is rapid, shunting into the inferior vena cava is likely. The needle is slightly withdrawn with subsequent slow injection of additional contrast. In the event of continued shunting of contrast despite needle withdrawal, one can reposition the needle or occlude the fistulous tract that

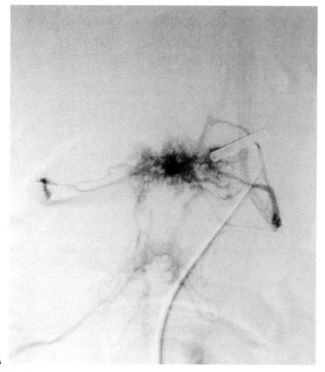
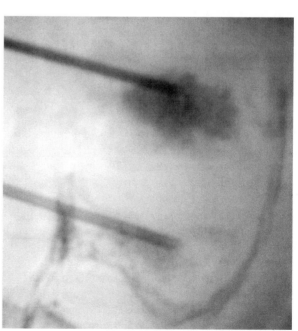

A   B

FIGURE 1–3 Vertebral body venography demonstrating filling of the vertebral body and segmental veins following injection of contrast dye in the **(A)** anteroposterior (AP) and **(B)** lateral planes. Drainage was deemed normal in this case.

has been created. Occlusion of the fistulae may be done with Gelfoam. Pledgets of Gelfoam soaked in contrast material are introduced via the needle. If positioning the Gelfoam is successful, injection of PMMA can proceed. Fistula blockage may also be accomplished by slow injection of thickened PMMA. If blockage of the fistula is successful, a second needle may then be inserted into the contralateral pedicle and injection of PMMA continued.

Preparation and introduction of PMMA is begun after positioning the needles and after vertebral venography has demonstrated appropriate venous outflow. The PMMA has two separate components: (1) methylmethacrylate polymer as a powder and (2) methylmethacrylate monomer as a liquid. The methylmethacrylate powder is placed in a 60-cc syringe from which 17 cc are measured and placed in each of two sterile plastic bowls. Three grams of sterile barium sulfate powder (E.Z.; EM, Inc.; Westbury, NY) is then added to each bowl to opacify the methylmethacrylate polymer. One must ensure that the methylmethacrylate polymer powder and the opacification material are mixed thoroughly before attempting to add methylmethacrylate monomer liquid. Next, 7 to 8 cc of the liquid monomer is added to the opacified polymer and mixed completely to a consistency of toothpaste. The thickened PMMA solution is poured into a 10-cc syringe. At this point, one may either load the PMMA into a commercial delivery device or opt to backload 1- or 3-cc syringes. The PMMA-filled delivery device is then attached to the syringe, and under intermittent fluoroscopic monitoring PMMA is injected in 0.5-cc aliquots (Fig. 1–4). Generally, it is possible to inject 5 to 10 cc of

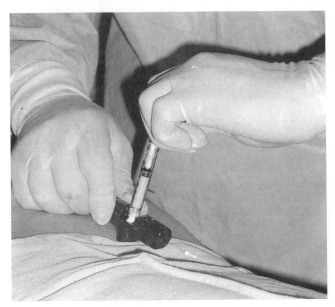

FIGURE 1–4 Injection of polymethylmethacrylate (PMMA) through the biopsy needle.

PMMA into each treated vertebral body. As injection of PMMA continues, it becomes progressively more difficult to add PMMA as it polymerizes and fills the vertebral body.

Whether to do unilateral or bilateral injection of PMMA, and the amount of PMMA needed to achieve adequate strength, are debatable. In osteoporotic vertebrae, near-complete to complete filling of the vertebral body may be accomplished with a unilateral injection of PMMA.[15] Often, a unilateral injection is all that is required. The dorsal concave portion of the vertebral body is not well visualized fluoroscopically; therefore, attempting to fill the entire vertebral body is not advised. This may cause extrusion of cement into the neural foramen or epidural space. If an initial injection resulted in opacification of only the lateral vertebral body, bilateral injection may prove useful. A significant correlation between pain relief and the amount of PMMA injected into a diseased vertebra has not been reported. An illustrative case is depicted in Fig. 1–5).

At the conclusion of the vertebroplasty procedure the needle is removed. Closure of the wound is usually unnecessary. Patients are kept recumbent for 2 hours and are then allowed to sit and ambulate with assistance. Patients are discharged on nonsteroidal antiinflammatory drugs (NSAIDs) and muscle relaxants later the same day. Ambulation is encouraged, and participation in activities of daily living is emphasized.

■ Vertebroplasty Complications

One of the most common complications following vertebroplasty is the development of radiculopathy. Acute radiculopathy has been reported to occur in up to 5% of cases. Symptoms may be transient and a short course of steroids may be helpful. In general, significant complications after vertebroplasty are low and occur in less than 10% of cases. Chiras et al[20] found a complication rate of 1.3% in osteoporotic compression fracture cases undergoing vertebroplasty; higher complication rates were noted with more destructive bone lesions such as hemangiomas (2.5%) and vertebral malignancies (10%). Cement leakage is a common problem associated with vertebroplasty and is reported to occur in 30 to 70% of cases; however, most instances of cement leakage are clinically inconsequential.[13]

Other complications of vertebroplasty include fractures of the rib or pedicle, pneumothorax, spinal cord compression, an increase in back pain, and infection. For immunocompromised patients or those with myeloma, tobramycin (1.2 g, Nebcin; Eli Lilly, Indianapolis, IN) is prophylactically added to the PMMA to help prevent infection. In addition, potential complications include soft tissue and intravenous extravasation of PMMA that may

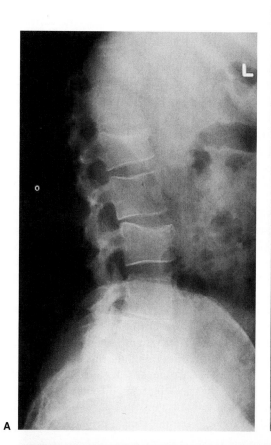

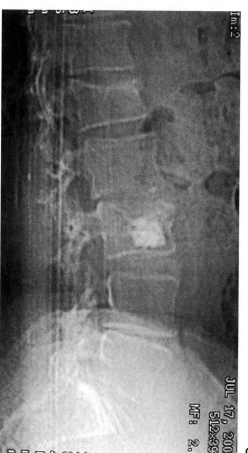

A

C

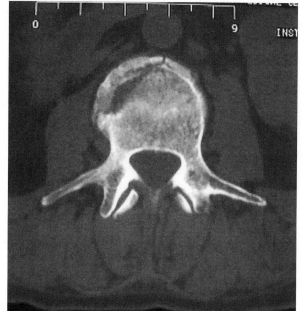

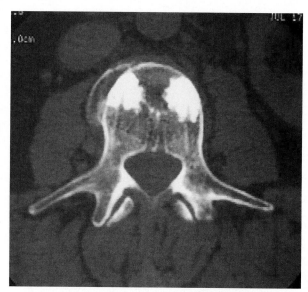

B

D

FIGURE 1–5 Case illustration. A 46-year-old man suffered traumatic compression fractures at L1 and L3. He complained of chronic back pain for several months following the injury, which was localizable to the L3 level. Lateral lumbosacral x-ray **(A)** and axial computed tomography (CT) scan **(B)** demonstrate the L3 fracture. He underwent vertebroplasty with bipedicular injection of PMMA. Lateral x-ray **(C)** and axial CT scan **(D)** show good placement of cement in the anterior third of the vertebral body.

result in pulmonary emboli. To avoid this, vertebral body venography is performed prior to injection of any PMMA. Alterations in the route and rate of PMMA delivery can be made following this assessment.

Fracture of adjacent vertebral levels following vertebroplasty does occur. The cause is most likely multifactorial: diffuse nature of the osteoporotic spine disease; relief of pain and rapid return to higher level of activity; increased strength in vertebrae that are subject to increased loads from kyphotic deformity. Gradual increase in activity and continued use of orthotic devices (for 6 weeks following vertebroplasty) may help prevent adjacent-level fracture in those at high risk.

■ Overview of Vertebroplasty

In practice, there are several controversial questions that are frequently raised about vertebroplasty. First, how many levels should be done in a patient with multiple compression fractures, and should adjacent levels be done prophylactically? Second, should the procedure be performed in the operating room (OR)? or in an interventional radiology suite? Third, is angiography necessary? Fourth, how much methyl is necessary to achieve the stated goals of pain relief and stability?

Although many patients present with multiple compression fractures, it is not always the case that all of them are causing pain, nor is it the case that all should have vertebroplasty performed on them. Bone scan and/or MRI may be helpful in distinguishing acute from old fractures and can be helpful in limiting the number of levels that require treatment. It is probably wise to remember in this patient population that it is best to treat the patient and not the x-rays. An argument can be made that treatment of multiple levels can reduce the degree of kyphosis and thus increase lung vital capacity. However, no data exist to support this hypothesis, and it is unlikely that kyphosis will be reduced in fractures more than 6 weeks old. Thus a focused approach designed to treat the symptomatic level(s), rather than an approach that treats every fracture, seems reasonable. An argument has also been made that adjacent levels should have prophylactic vertebroplasty performed because acutely increasing the strength of one vertebral body puts adjacent levels at increased risk for fracture. However, once again, no data exist to support adjacent-level fracture at a rate above that for normal vertebrae.

Whether the procedure should be performed in the OR or in an interventional radiology suite depends on the facilities available at individual institutions. Ideally, the procedure should be performed by an experienced physician who has biplanar imaging available, sterile surgical conditions, and the ability to immediately proceed with a decompressive procedure in the event of cement extrusion into the spinal canal. Thus the ideal location would be in an OR with biplanar imaging. A single fluoroscope can be used, but the necessity to continuously alternate between AP and lateral views is technically unsatisfactory. In the absence of the ideal, an interventional radiology suite is acceptable if immediate access to an operating room is available.

Vertebral angiography, although not absolutely necessary, is highly recommended. It confirms needle-tip placement and tests the rate of venous efflux from the vertebral body. In our experience, we reposition the needle tip or otherwise modify our injection technique ~30% of the time based on the information provided by the angiogram.

Finally, no data exist at this time that absolutely dictate the amount of methyl that should be injected. Some data suggest that pain is alleviated with 3 cc of methyl as effectively as with larger volumes. However, it is not likely that 3 cc of methyl achieves the goal of vertebral stability. Thus, if stability is also a desired goal, it seems rational that volumes that more adequately fill the vertebral body would be necessary. However, larger volumes require very close scrutiny under biplanar fluoroscopy to avoid cement extrusion. Thus "risk vs. benefit" must be closely assessed in each individual patient.

■ Indications for Kyphoplasty

Indications for kyphoplasty are identical to those for vertebroplasty, but the goals of the two procedures differ. Vertebroplasty makes no attempt to restore the vertebra to normal height or correct any kyphotic deformities, whereas kyphoplasty attempts to restore vertebral height, reduce kyphophotic deformity, and improve the safety of PMMA injection. A major limitation of vertebroplasty is extrusion of cement into the spinal canal and neural foramen. The rate of cement extravasation has been reported to be as high as 30% when used to treat osteoporotic compression fractures.[15] Treatment of metastases is associated with even higher rates of cement extravasation; 65% of patients in one series experienced some degree of cement extrusion.[21] During vertebroplasty, the cement is forced into an unexpanded matrix of cancellous bone, creating a high-pressure environment that increases risk of leakage. In contrast, during kyphoplasty, the cement slowly fills an already-expanded cavity; there is less pressure required for the injection and therefore risk of cement leakage may be decreased.

■ Kyphoplasty Procedure

Kyphoplasty is a procedure whereby a bone tamp or balloon is inserted into the vertebral body. The goal of the procedure is restoring the vertebral body back to its original height and creating a cavity within the bone that may be filled with bone cement.[22,23] Expansion of the vertebral body is followed radiographically by placing contrast medium in the balloon. Usually two balloons are used when doing kyphoplasty procedures.

The kyphoplasty procedure, as first described by Garfin and coworkers,[22] is summarized below. Placement of the bone tamp is done via a transpedicular or an extrapedicular approach. This is accomplished with the aid of a guide pin and biplanar fluoroscopy. Once cannulation of the vertebral body has occurred, an obturator is passed over the guidewire and inserted into the vertebral body. Additionally, a working cannula is passed over the obturator until the cannula tip is in the posterior portion of the vertebral body. The inflatable tamp is passed through a corridor created by drilling along the cannula path. After this, the device is inflated under fluoroscopic guidance to a pressure of no more than 220 psi. Balloon pressure monitoring is accomplished with the use of an in-line pressure gauge. Once a sufficiently sized cavity has been formed and the maximum allowable reduction has been obtained, PMMA cement is mixed with barium. At this point, smaller cannulas filled with cement are inserted into the working cannula. The cement is allowed to thicken prior to its application; this is determined by repeat suspension of a 2-cm^3 bolus from a spatula until it is observed that cement does not fall from the spatula. At this point, the viscosity of the cement is considered sufficient to permit injection.

The cement-filled cannula is inserted into the working cannula, with subsequent passage into the anterior vertebral body wall. A plunger-like effect is obtained by using a stainless steel stylet to extrude the cement into its target location. Filling the cavity with cement continues under lateral fluoroscopic guidance and ceases when a mantle of cement reaches back about two thirds to the cortex of the posterior portion of the vertebral body.

■ Kyphoplasty Complications

No complications related to balloon tamps have been reported during kyphoplasty procedures.[22,23] Several complications, all related in some way to needle insertion, have been documented. During phase I testing of an inflatable bone tamp, Lieberman et al[23] found that kyphoplasty was a safe procedure; they had no significant complications related to their device. Cement extravasation was the most common problem occurring in 8.6% of their patients. There were no clinical sequelae resulting from cement extravasation. Additionally, the authors were encouraged that rates of cement extravasation during their kyphoplasty procedure were lower than those of published vertebroplasty series.

■ Overview of Kyphoplasty

Just as with vertebroplasty, questions have been raised about kyphoplasty. Specifically, can kyphoplasty realistically achieve reduction of the fracture? Is it logical to assume that filling a created hole within the vertebral body will confer stability on the vertebral body? Finally, is there an improved clinical outcome to justify the additional cost?

Theoretically, inflating a balloon against closely adjacent end plates following a fracture should achieve some reduction of the fracture. However, minimal data exist to support this in reality. Logically, because the natural history of a fracture is to heal, and because experience with long-bone fracture suggests that reduction becomes extremely difficult sometime between 3 and 6 weeks following the fracture, it seems likely that attempts at reduction after 6 weeks of medical treatment would be met with a high probability of reduction failure. Because the current recommendations for kyphoplasty (or vertebroplasty) are to proceed only after a 6-week to 3-month trial of medical treatment fails, it would seem that the ability of either to achieve significant reduction of kyphosis is quite small.

The second question that has been raised is regarding the philosophy of filling the interstices of the vertebral body versus filling the cavity created by the balloon expansion. In the case where the vertebral collapse is great enough that the balloon contacts both end plates during expansion, a solid column would be created by filling the cavity with methyl. However, if the collapse is not that great, then filling the cavity would achieve only filling a gap that was created by the balloon and that would be surrounded by cancellous bone. This would most likely not achieve stability. In that case, filling the interstices of the cancellous bone would seem to be advantageous and more likely to create a stable construct than just filling a previously created defect.

Finally, the cost of kyphoplasty is significantly greater than vertebroplasty. To justify the additional cost, one or more of several criteria should be met. Kyphoplasty should (1) provide greater stability, (2) provide better pain relief, (3) be safer, or (4) be easier to perform in a shorter time period. Most studies suggest equivalent results in stability and pain relief and in complication rates. Furthermore, both procedures utilize a similar basic technique and seem roughly equivalent in ease/difficulty. Thus it is reasonable to question the cost/benefit ratio of the kyphoplasty procedure.

■ Conclusions

Vertebroplasty can reduce pain in 90 to 95% of patients suffering osteoporotic vertebral fractures.[12,13,24] Additionally, improvements are made in mobility and in activities of daily living. Also of note, patients who have undergone percutaneous vertebroplasty decrease their use of narcotic pain medications. Kyphoplasty is a new addition for the treatment of compression fractions that may offer restoration of vertebral height, kyphotic deformity correction, as well as pain relief. The procedures are associated with acceptable complication rates that, it is hoped, will be further reduced with increasing clinical experiences. Future work on the timing of procedures, prophylactic treatment of adjacent levels, and long-term clinical outcomes will help guide and popularize implementation of these beneficial, minimally invasive techniques.

REFERENCES

1. Kado DM, Browner WS, Palmero L, Nevitt MC, Genant HK, Cummings SR. Vertebral fractures and mortality in older women: a prospective study. Study of Osteoporotic Fractures Research Group. Arch Intern Med 1999;159:1215–1220

2. Lyles KW. Management of patients with vertebral compression fractures. Pharmacotherapy 1999;19:21S–24S

3. Cooper C, Atkinson EJ, Jacobsen SJ, O'Fallon WM, Melton LJ III. Incidence of clinically diagnosed vertebral fractures: a population-based study in Rochester, Minnesota, 1985–1989. J Bone Miner Res 1993;7:221–227

4. Melton LJ III. Epidemiology of spinal osteoporosis. Spine 1997; 22(24 suppl):2S–11S

5. Riggs BL, Melton LJ III. Involutional osteoporosis. N Engl J Med 1986;314:1676–1686

6. Silverman SL. The clinical consequences of vertebral compression fractures. Bone 1992;13:527–531

7. Cook DJ, Guyatt GH, Adachi JD, et al. Quality of life issues in women with vertebral fractures due to osteoporosis. Arthritis Rheum 1993;36:750–756

8. Gold DT. The clinical impact of vertebral fractures: quality of life in women with osteoporosis. Bone 1996;18(suppl):1897–1904

9. Schlaich C, Minnie HW, Bruckner T, et al. Reduced pulmonary function in patients with spinal osteoporotic fractures. Osteoporos Int 1998;8:261–267

10. Convertino VA, Bloomfield SA, Greenleaf JF. An overview of the issues: physiological effects of bed rest and restricted physical activity. Med Sci Sports Exerc 1997;29:187–190

11. Uthoff HK, Jaworski ZF. Bone loss in response in response to long term immoblization. J Bone Joint Surg Br 1978;60:420–429

12. Barr JD, Barr MS, Lemley TJ, McCann RM. Percutaneous vertebroplasty for pain relief and spinal stabilization. Spine 2000;25:923–928

13. Cortet B, Cotton A, Boutry N, et al. Percutaneous vertebroplasty in the treatment of osteoporotic vertebral compression fractures: an open prospective study. J Rheumatol 1999;26:2222–2228

14. Cyteval C, Sarrabere M, Roux JO, et al. Acute osteoporotic vertebral collapse: open study on percutaneous injection of acrylic surgical cement in 20 patients. AJR Am J Roentgenol 1999;173:1685–1690

15. Jensen ME, Evans AJ, Mathis JM, Kallmes DF, Cloft HJ, Dion JE. Percutaneous polymethylmethacrylate vertebroplasty in the treatment of osteoporotic vertebral body compression fractures: technical aspects. AJNR Am J Neuroradiol 1997;18:1897–1904

16. Belkoff SM, Maroney M, Fenton DC, Mathis JM. An in vitro biochemical evaluation evaluation of bone cements used in percutaneous vertebroplasty. Bone 1999;25(2 suppl):23S–26S

17. Tohmeh AG, Mathis JM, Fenton DC, Levine AM, Belkoff SM. Biochemical efficacy of unipedicular versus bipedicular vertebroplasty for the management of osteoporotic compression fractures. Spine 1999;24:1772–1776

18. Galibert P. Note Préliminaire sur le traitement des angiomas vertébraux par vertebroplastie acrylique percutanée. Neurochirurgie 1987;33:166–167

19. Lapras J, Mottolese C, Deruty R, et al. Injetion percutané de methylmétacrylate dans le traitement de l'oestéoporose et ostélyse vertébrale grave. Ann Chir 1987;43:371–375

20. Chiras J, Depriester C, Weill A, Sola-Martinez MT, Deramond H. Vertebroplasties percutenées: technique et indications. J Neuroradiol 1997;24:45–59

21. Weill A, Chiras J, Simon JM, Rose M, Sola-Martinez T, Enkaoua E. Spinal metastases: indications for and results of percutaneous injection of acrylic cement. Radiology 1996;199:241–247

22. Garfin SR, Yuan HA, Reiley MA. Kyphoplasty and vertebroplasty for the treatment of painful osteoporotic compression fractures. Spine 2001;26:1511–1515

23. Lieberman IH, Dudeney S, Reinhardt M-K, Bell G. Initial outcome and efficacy of kyphoplasty in the treatment of painful osteoporotic vertebral compression fractures. Spine 2001;26:1631–1638

24. Deramond H, Depriester C, Galipert P, Le Gars D. Percutaneous vertebroplasty with polymethylmethacrylate: technique, indications, and results. Radiol Clin North Am 1998;36:533–546

2

Mechanisms of Pain Relief Following Vertebroplasty and Kyphoplasty

LISA L. GUYOT, RAJU BALAHADRA, AND RICHARD D. FESSLER

Objectives: On completion of this chapter, the reader should be able to discuss potential mechanisms of pain relief achieved through vertebroplasty and/or kyphoplasty.

Accreditation: The American Association of Neurological Surgeons is accredited by the Accreditation Council for Continuing Medical Education to sponsor continuing medical education for physicians.

Credit: The American Association of Neurological Surgeons designates this continuing medical education activity for a maximum of 15 credits in Category I of the Physician's Recognition Award of the American Medical Association.

The Home Study Examination is online at www.aans.org/education/books/vertebro.asp

Vertebroplasty was first utilized in 1987 to treat a painful vertebral body hemangioma.[1] Since that time, its uses have expanded to include treatment of painful osteoporotic and steroid-induced compression fractures[2–6] and metastatic disease of the spine.[7,8] Vertebroplasty has been particularly useful in treating the pain associated with osteoporotic compression fractures. In properly selected patients, authors report a 90 to 95% reduction in pain.[2,4,9,10] More recently, kyphoplasty, a vertebroplasty variation that utilizes a percutaneously placed balloon to elevate fractured end plates and fill the resulting void with methylmethacrylate, has also been shown to reduce pain. In addition, kyphoplasty theoretically provides the added benefit of fracture reduction.[11,12] Despite tremendous clinical success, the mechanism of pain relief following vertebroplasty and kyphoplasty is unknown. This chapter describes the pain pathways of the spine and offers several possible means by which vertebroplasty and kyphoplasty relieve pain.

■ Innervation of the Spine and Soft Tissue

The spine can be divided generally into anterior and posterior elements when describing innervation. The anterior elements include the ventral dura, intervertebral disk,

posterior longitudinal ligament (PLL), vertebral body, anterior longitudinal ligament (ALL), and prevertebral muscles (psoas major, psoas minor, quadratus lumborum, and lateral intertransverse muscles). The posterior elements include the lamina, facet joints and capsules, ligamentum flavum, supraspinous and interspinous ligaments, and intrinsic back muscles. The anterior elements are supplied by nerves arising from the ventral rami of the spinal nerves, and the posterior elements are innervated by medial branches of the dorsal rami of the spinal nerves (Fig. 2–1). Nociceptive fibers penetrate the outer third of the annulus fibrosus. Nerves to the outer disk arise directly from the origin of the ventral ramus. Other branches to the lateral and anterior disk arise from the rami communicantes. Nerves tend to distribute to disks at the same level or occasionally the level below.

The posterior annulus, the PLL, the anterior dural sac, and the blood vessels of the anterior spine are innervated by branches of the sinuvertebral nerve. The sinuvertebral nerve is formed by the union of a nerve branch from the origin of the ventral ramus and an autonomic root from the gray ramus communicans.[13] Interestingly, a recent report by Chandler et al, showed that anesthetic blockade of the gray rami communicans resulted in relief of pain in patients with vertebral compression fractures secondary to osteoporosis. The PLL is also well innervated by both complex encapsulated and

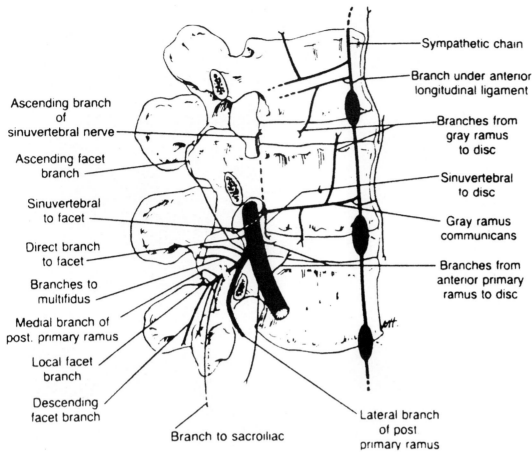

FIGURE 2–1 Segmental innervation of the lumbar spine. Disk innervation: Branches from the sympathetic chain innervate the lateral and anterior portions of the disk above and below. The recurrent sinuvertebral nerve, which is formed from the gray ramus communicans and mixed spinal nerves, innervates the posterior and posterolateral portions of the disk at two levels inside the spinal canal. The ventral ramus sends small branches to the disk at the level of nerve exit. Facet and erector spinae muscles: The posterior primary ramus sends medial branches to the facet at the level of nerve exit and to the facet below. According to some investigators there is also a branch to the facet above (as shown). There are also medial branches to multifidus muscle. The intermediate erector spinae muscle (longissimus) is innervated by the intermediate branches of posterior primary rami. Lateral erector spinae (iliocostalis) is innervated by the lateral branches of posterior primary rami, which also innervate cutaneous tissue.

poorly myelinated free nerve endings. In a series of over 700 lumbar laminectomies done under local anesthesia, Kulisch et al. determined that stimulation of the PLL and the outer layer of the annulus fibrosus caused the most subjective low back pain. This suggests that deformation or stretching of the PLL in compression fractures may be a significant source of back pain. Innervation of the ALL arises from the gray rami communicans (postganglionic sympathetics that travel with the spinal nerves to innervate the blood vessels, smooth muscles, and sweat glands of the skin) or by a branch from the sympathetic chain.[16]

The facet joints and the supraspinous and interspinous ligaments are supplied by medial branches of the dorsal rami of the spinal nerves. The facet joints are innervated by the medial branch of the dorsal ramus from the branch exiting at the level and the segment above.

The facet joint and the supraspinous and interspinous ligaments contain free and encapsulated nerve endings that, if stimulated, can cause back pain.[17]

The intrinsic back muscles are supplied in a segmental fashion by the lateral branches of the dorsal rami of the spinal nerves.[16]

■ Possible Mechanisms of Pain Relief

Improved Load-Bearing

In properly selected patients, vertebroplasty and kyphoplasty produce substantial pain relief within minutes to hours following the procedure. Pain pathways in the surrounding tissue appear to be altered in response to mechanical, chemical, vascular, and thermal stimuli after

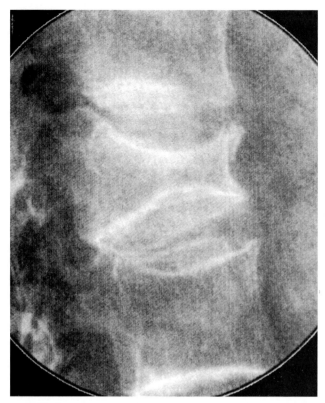

FIGURE 2–2 A lateral radiograph of a vertebral compression fracture secondary to osteoporosis. Bilateral transpedicular placement of vertebral balloons has been performed.

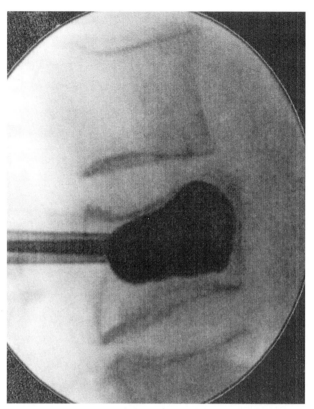

FIGURE 2–3 A lateral radiograph following inflation of the kyphoplasty balloons. Note the elevation of the end plates and the size of the potential bone void created for delivery of polymethylmethacrylate after deflation and removal of the balloons.

the injection of polymethylmethacrylate (PMMA), with resultant pain relief. Vertebroplasty and kyphoplasty restore mechanical strength to osteoporotic bone. In fact, even minimal amounts of PMMA appear able to improve bone strength.[18,19] Methylmethacrylate augmentation reduces vertebral body compliance to flexion/extension by 23% and lateral bending by 26%. The improved load-bearing ability and mechanical stabilization may reduce micromotion of the vertebral body and improve bone axial load-bearing capability. The improved stability and strength of the motion segment are hypothesized to reduce the pain stimulus.[7]

Fracture Reduction

Kyphoplasty is performed by placing bilateral vertebral body balloons into the fractured vertebrae (Fig. **2–2**). The balloons are inflated sequentially over several minutes under fluoroscopic guidance. In theory, balloon inflation elevates fractured end plates (Fig. **2–3**). The balloons also create a potential space within the vertebral body into which methylmethacrylate is delivered. Kyphoplasty appears to provide the load-bearing benefits of vertebroplasty with the added potential benefit of fracture reduction. Fracture reduction may result in

restoration of the PLL and ALL to a more favorable anatomic position, with a resultant decline in pain from pain afferents.

Direct Tissue Toxicity

Polymethylmethacrylate monomer is an organic solvent. Exposure of tissue to unreacted monomer is directly toxic to cells.[19] Exposure of pain afferents within the vertebral body to unreacted PMMA may result in direct damage to nerve endings with resultant diminished pain perception. This may also explain in part the effectiveness of vertebroplasty in local tumor control in terms of tumor necrosis. The ratio of monomer to powder during preparation, as well as the addition of an antibiotic, can affect the relative degree of tissue toxicity.[20]

Thermal Injury

Polymerization of PMMA is an exothermic reaction. Temperatures as high as 50° to 57°C have been recorded at the bone–cement interface during polymerization of PMMA.[20] Temperatures of 42° to 47°C are sufficient to destroy several types of cells. Tissue cells known to be susceptible to thermal injury at these temperatures include cartilage, embryonal tumors, and carcinoma cells.[21] Following vertebroplasty and kyphoplasty, PMMA curing and the subsequent elevations in local temperature may play a role in pain relief through thermal injury to free nerve endings. In addition, in cases of metastatic spine disease, the elevated temperatures result in destruction of tumor cells, and PMMA physically alters vascular supply. Thermal injury, reduction of vascular supply to tumors, and direct tumor thermal injury are all possible mechanisms of pain relief following use of PMMA.

■ Conclusion

Vertebroplasty and kyphoplasty have been shown to be clinically effective therapies for pathologic compression fractures due to osteoporosis, metastatic tumors, and aggressive hemangiomas. Although the exact mechanism for their effectiveness is unknown, it likely involves a combination of effects. Polymethylmethacrylate improves the load-bearing ability of bone and may directly interfere with pain afferents through direct tissue toxicity and thermal injury. In addition, kyphoplasty provides an element of fracture reduction with potential return of more normal ligamentous morphology. In cases of spinal metastases, PMMA injection (in addition to mechanically stabilizing the vertebral body) may also lead to coagulation of the tumor vascular supply and direct toxic effects on the tumor, thereby reducing the tumor load.

REFERENCES

1. Gailbert P, Deramond H, Rosat P, LeGars D. Preliminary note on the treatment of vertebral angioma by percutaneous acrylic vertebroplasty. Neurochirurgie 1987;33:166–168
2. Barr JD, Barr MS, Lemley TJ, McCann RM. Percutaneous vertebroplasty for pain relief and spinal stabilization. Spine 2000;25:923–928
3. Cyteval C, Sarrabere MPB, Roux JO, et al. Acute osteoporotic vertebral collapse: open study on percutaneous injection of acrylic surgical cement in 20 patients. AJR Am J Roentgenol 1999;173:1685–1690
4. Cortet B, Cotton A, Boutry N, et al. Percutaneous vertebroplasty in the treatment of osteoporotic vertebral compression fractures: an open prospective study. J Rheumatol 1999;26:2222–2228
5. Jensen ME, Evans AJ, Mathis JM, Kallmes DF, Cloft HJ, Dion JE. Percutaneous polymethylmethacrylate vertebroplasty in the treatment of osteoporotic vertebral body compression fractures: technical aspects. AJNR Am J Neuroradiol 1997;18:1897–1904
6. Mathis JM, Petri M, Naff N. Percutaneous vertebroplasty treatment of steroid-induced osteoporotic compression fractures. Arthritis Rheum 1998;41:171–175
7. Guelbenzu S, Gomez J, Garcia-Asensio S, Barrena R, Ferrandez D. Preoperative percutaneous vertebroplasty in hemangioma compression. Rev Neurol 1999;28:397–400
8. Ide C, Gangi A, Rimmelin A, et al. Vertebral hemangiomas with spinal cord compression: the place of preoperative percutaneous vertebroplasty with methylmethacrylate. Neuroradiology 1996;38:585–589
9. Dousset V, Mousselard H, de Monck d'User L, et al. Asymptomatic cervical haemangioma treated by percutaneous vertebroplasty. Neuroradiology 1996;38:392–394
10. Feydy A, Cognard C, Miaux Y, et al. Acrylic vertebroplasty in symptomatic cervical vertebral haemangiomas: report of 2 cases. Neuroradiology 1996;38:389–391
11. Gailbert P, Deramond H. Percutaneous acrylic vertebroplasty as a treatment of vertebral angioma as well as painful and debilitating diseases. Chirurgie 1990;116:326–324
12. Weill A, Chiras J, Simon JM, Rose M, Sola-Martinez T, Enkaoua E. Spinal metastases: indications for and results of percutaneous injection of acrylic surgical cement. Radiology 1996;199:241–247
13. Kaemmerlen P, Thiesse P, Bouvard H, Biron P, Mornex F, Jonas P. Percutaneous vertebroplasty in the treatment of metasteses: technique and results. J Radiol 1989;70:557–562
14. Cardon T, Hachulla E, Flipo RM, et al. Percutaneous vertebroplasty with acrylic cement in the treatment of a Langerhans' cell vertebral histiocytosis. Clin Rheumatol 1994;13:518–521
15. Cortet B, Cotton A, Boutry N, et al. Percutaneous vertebroplasty in patients with osteolytic metastases or multiple myeloma. Rev Rhum Engl Ed 1997;64:177–183
16. Wilson DR, Myers ER, Mathis JM, et al. Effect of augmentation on the mechanics of vertebral wedge fractures. Spine 2000;25:158–165
17. Belkoff SM, Maroney M, Fenton DC, Mathis JM. An in vitro biomechanical evaluation of bone cements used in percutaneous vertebroplasty. Bone 1999;25(2 Suppl):23S–26S
18. Tohmeh AG, Mathis JM, Fenton DC, Levine AM, Belkoff SM. Biomechanical efficacy of unipedicular versus bipedicular vertebroplasty for the management of osteoporotic compression fractures. Spine 1999;24:1772–1776
19. Dean JR, Ison KT, Gishen P. The strengthening effect of percutaneous vertebroplasty. Clin Radiol 2000;55:471–476
20. Lyles KW. Management of patients with vertebral compression fractures. Pharmacotherapy 1999;19:21S–24S
21. Melton LJ III. Epidemiology of spinal osteoporosis. Spine 1997;22(24 suppl):2S–11S

3

Anatomic Constraints and Concerns of Vertebroplasty and Kyphoplasty

MARCELO A. RODRIGUES, ROBERT Q. INGRAHAM, AND T. GLENN PAIT

Objectives: On completion of this chapter, the reader should be able to describe the relevant anatomical features of the vertebral body as they relate to vertebroplasty and kyphoplasty.

Accreditation: The American Association of Neurological Surgeons is accredited by the Accreditation Council for Continuing Medical Education to sponsor continuing medical education for physicians.

Credit: The American Association of Neurological Surgeons designates this continuing medical education activity for a maximum of 15 credits in Category I of the Physician's Recognition Award of the American Medical Association.

The Home Study Examination is online at www.aans.org/education/books/vertebro.asp

The term *vertebroplasty* originally defined an open surgical procedure in which bone graft or surgical cement was introduced as a replacement of the vertebral body to mechanically improve bone strength.[1] Today vertebroplasty can be defined as "a procedure in which polymethylmethacrylate (PMMA) is injected into a vertebral body compression fracture."[2] This procedure can be performed percutaneously with computed tomography (CT) guidance or direct fluoroscopic visualization, or as an open surgical procedure. An appreciation of anatomic structures and variants of normal may help to improve the results of vertebroplasty.

Since Galibert et al[3] injected PMMA using a percutaneous procedure into a C2 vertebra that had been destroyed by an aggressive hemangioma, vertebroplasty has been the subject of several studies to improve the quality of life of patients whose underlying disease required improved management or adjuvant therapies.[1-12]

The interest in percutaneous vertebroplasty has continued to grow after its introduction into the United States in 1994. The main indication of percutaneous vertebroplasty is pain caused by vertebral compression fractures resulting from either osteoporosis or tumor infiltration.[1,4,7-9] The most common lesions are caused by osteoporosis that may be age related (primary) or due to steroid use (secondary).[4,9] The most common tumor infiltrations are those caused by osteolytic metastases or multiple myeloma. Other pathologic fractures include compressions due to aggressive hemangiomas and giant cell tumors. The goal of the operation is to bring about stability to a mechanically unstable vertebral body, thus relieving the patient's pain. Several mechanisms have been put forth to explain the pain relief, including thermal necrosis and chemotoxicity of the intraosseous pain receptors, as well as ischemia, which may result from the mass of the bone cement or occlusion of tumor vessels.[1,4,7]

The technique is based on a transpedicular approach to the vertebral body to fill it with PMMA as described by Gangi et al.[7] The patient is placed in a prone position, and under fluoroscopy or CT scan important anatomic structures are localized.

Understanding key anatomic structures of the vertebrae may be quite helpful during vertebroplasty treatment. Bony parameters should be measured before and during the procedure to avoid mishaps such as pedicle penetration and adjacent structure damage.

■ Results and Complications

There is no medical procedure without risks and benefits. Although new techniques to guide the physician and surgeon are improving geometrically, problems can occur. Fevers, transient worsening of pain, radiculopathy,

14

rib fractures, PMMA pulmonary embolism, transient dysphasia, infection, and lack of pain relief have all been reported.[1–12] Due to the intimate relations between the vertebrae and structures such as the pleura, lungs, aorta, esophagus, thoracic duct, sympathetic chain, vena cava, azygos vein, intercostal vessels, and neural structures, problems arise even for the most experienced practitioner.

Jensen et al[1] reported 90% pain relief in 29 patients with osteoporotic fractures. Two patients related pain relief immediately after vertebroplasty. In another study, Barr et al[8] reported 38 patients treated for osteoporotic fractures in which 63% had marked to complete pain relief, 32% moderate relief, and 5% no significant change. Barr's group further reported a 50% significant pain relief for malignant lesions. Other researchers described 90 to 100% pain relief for treatment of osteoporotic fractures.[3–6] Weill and his group[14] reported clear improvement of pain in 73% of the 37 patients with 52 metastatic lesions. Cotton et al[9] also reported the treatment of 40 metastatic lesions in 37 patients with 59% marked pain relief. Thus vertebroplasty and such procedures can indeed provide avenues of benefit for certain patients.

■ Vertebral Anatomy

During the last 20 years many studies about the bony dimensions of the individual vertebral structures have been extensively reported. These works describe in detail the shapes and sizes of the various components of the spine. Surgical techniques for spinal instrumentation spawned the need for anatomic studies about the vertebral anatomy.[15–62]

For the posterior approach the pedicle is the most important structure for reaching the vertebral body, thus avoiding the neural and other vital structures. The articular facet, pars interarticularis, lamina, vertebral body, spinous process, and transverse process also have important significance in surgical approaches.

Surgical anatomic researchers often use cadavers and CT measurements to perform their studies. The tools most employed in cadaveric studies are calipers and goniometers with an accuracy of 1 mm and 1 degree, respectively. Axial, sagittal, and coronal measurements are recorded.

■ Thoracic Anatomy

Thoracic anatomy has been reported extensively due to new techniques of spinal fixation and stabilization. The main reason for this variety of studies is the potential for injury, which may occur in the thoracic region during pedicle screw placement or pedicle manipulation from percutaneous procedures. The mediolateral dimension

of the pedicle and its relation to the epidural space are relatively small. This lends itself to increased difficulty with any procedure in this region. The close relation among vital structures such as the aorta, lungs, vena cava, esophagus, and neural elements also contributes to excessive care needed in this area.

Panjabi et al[45] has described one quantitative three-dimensional anatomic study with 12 fresh autopsy specimens. Vaccaro et al[55,56] used CT scans to evaluate 19 thoracic spines in living patients with no evidence of any vertebral deformity and in 17 human cadavers to define these parameters. McCormack et al[39] measured the pedicular anatomy in 11 cadavers and Ebraheim et al[25] used 43 dry thoracic specimens to obtain their data. Zindrick et al[62] compared specimens in two ways: postmortem adult spine specimens with direct measurement and posterior roentgenography and computerized axial tomographic measurements. Scoles et al[53] studied 50 normal adult vertebral columns postmortem.

■ Thoracic Vertebral Body

The vertebral body shows a diameter slightly greater in its anteroposterior aspect than its transverse dimension. The lateral and ventral surfaces are concave. The first thoracic vertebra is a transitional vertebra, and its body resembles the seventh cervical vertebra.[19,20,29,30,42,54]

In Panjabi et al's[45] study, the vertebral body height showed a gradual increase from 14.1 mm at T1 to 22.7 mm at T12, an increase of almost 60%. This corresponds to an average increase of 0.8 mm per vertebrae. The height of the vertebral body was measured taking the distance between two parallel lines at the superior and inferior end plates[45] (Table 3–1).

Scoles et al[53] reported significant difference by gender. The average vertebral body height was 1 mm greater per level in the male population. Their results also showed a height increase from 16.8 mm at T1 to 25.9 mm at T12 corresponding to Panjabi's report of an increase of almost 0.8 mm per vertebral level[45,53] (Table 3–1).

TABLE 3–1 Thoracic Anatomy: Body Height

	Punjabi	*Scoles*
T1	14.1	16.8
T2	15.6	
T3	15.7	18.6
T4	16.2	
T5	16.2	
T6	17.4	19.8
T7	18.2	
T8	18.7	
T9	19.3	21.8
T10	20.2	
T11	21.3	
T12	22.7	25.9

TABLE 3–2 Thoracic Anatomy: Body Anteroposterior Diameter (mm)

	Punjabi	Scoles
T1	18.5	15.5
T2	19.6	
T3	22.7	18.7
T4	23.3	
T5	24.3	
T6	26.0	23.7
T7	27.4	
T8	27.9	
T9	29.3	27.4
T10	30.5	
T11	31.9	
T12	32.8	28.8

The anteroposterior diameter of the vertebral body was measured as a unique dimension by some authors, whereas others used two dimensions related to both end plates (superior and inferior).[45] Relative differences between male and female anatomy were found except at T1. Scoles et al reported a gradual increase from 15.5 mm at T1 to 28.8 mm at T12, an average almost 2 mm smaller than Panjabi's[45,53] (Table **3–2**).

Panjabi et al[45] also reported an increase from T1 to T12 ranging 55% for the lower end plate to 73% for the upper end plate. They found values of 18.5 mm at T1 to 32.8 mm at T12 (Table **3–2**).

There was no significant difference for the transverse vertebral body diameters. The width of the thoracic vertebral body ranged from 14.5 mm at T1 to 41.7 mm at T12. The transverse vertebra body diameter ranges almost 2 mm greater in the male population[45,53] (Table **3–3**).

A significant and constant increase was found in all dimensions of the vertebral body from T1 to T12, ranging from 50 to 60% caudally.[45,53]

■ Thoracic Pedicle

The pedicles of the thoracic vertebrae are directed dorsally starting at the vertebral body and ending at the lamina. They are oval and directed slightly laterally and upward.[19,20,30,31,42,50,54,59]

TABLE 3–3 Thoracic Anatomy: Body Width

	Punjabi	Scoles
T1	24.5	26.4
T2	24.9	
T3	24.6	27.6
T4	24.5	
T5	24.9	
T6	26.2	28.7
T7	27.8	
T8	29.5	
T9	30.6	32.5
T10	31.9	
T11	34.9	
T12	39.0	41.7

TABLE 3–4 Thoracic Anatomy: Interpedicular Distance

	McCormack	Scoles	Punjabi	Ebraheim	Berry
T1	20.6	21.2	21.8	14.4	
T2	20.0		19.5	15.5	18.1
T3	18.9	17.4	18.3	17.0	
T4	17.8		17.0	17.5	
T5	18.0		17.1	15.0	
T6	17.9	16.5	17.3	15.2	
T7	18.3		17.3	160	17.2
T8	18.7		17.7	16.0	
T9	1901	16.8	17.9	165	
T10	19.8		18.2	16.0	
T11	21.0		19.4	18.0	
T12	20.5	19.9	22.2	20.0	20.5

Interpedicular Distance

The interpedicular distance was measured between right and left pedicles in its shortest distance. There were no significant differences among the interpedicular distances. The findings showed that the narrowest space was usually in the midthoracic region T4-T6 (15 mm to 17.3 mm). The widest distance was found at the rostral and caudal ends of the thoracic region T1 and T12 (20.6 mm to 22.2 mm). The results of five important studies are shown[18,23,39,45,53] (Table **3–4**).

Pedicle Width

The linear measurement was done in all cases by taking the shortest point of the pedicle width. Pedicle width was the shortest in the midthoracic region. Significant variation was found among this measurement in several studies. The results shown by Vaccaro and Scoles were consistently smaller than those reported by Panjabi, McCormack, Zindrick, and Ebraheim[25,39,45,53,55,62] (Table **3–5**).

On average, McCormack showed sizes 2.4 mm larger than reports by Panjabi, Ebraheim, and Zindrick, but with no significant statistic difference.[25,39,45,62] In all studies no significant difference was found between both sides. Gender also showed no significant difference. Although these authors used different measurement techniques, the results were similar. The tendency is for

TABLE 3–5 Thoracic Anatomy: Pedicle Width

	Vaccaro	Zindrick	McCormick	Scoles	Panjabi	Ebraheim
T1		7.9	8.3	7.3	8.2	8.8
T2		7.0	9.2		8.4	6.0
T3		5.6	9.5	3.9	7.0	4.1
T4	4.5	4.7	9.1		5.5	3.9
T5	4.4	4.5	9.7		6.2	4.6
T6	4.6	5.2	9.3	3.5	6.0	3.6
T7	4.9	5.3	8.8		6.5	4.5
T8	5.1	5.9	9.4		6.7	5.0
T9	5.8	6.1	10.8	3.9	7.6	5.3
T10	6.7	6.3	11.0		8.3	5.6
T11	8.0	7.8	10.7		8.8	8.3
T12	7.8	7.1	11.1	7.4	8.8	8.0

TABLE 3–6 Thoracic Anatomy: Pedicle Height

	Vaccaro	Zindrick	McCormick	Scoles	Panjabi
T1		9.9	8.4	9.2	9.3
T2		12.0	10.7		11.1
T3		12.4	11.8	11.8	11.8
T4	10.1	12.1	12.5		11.9
T5	10.0	11.9	13.1		11.2
T6	10.1	12.2	11.2	11.5	12.2
T7	10.8	12.1	12.2		11.8
T8	11.1	12.8	13.7		12.5
T9	12.3	13.8	14.0	12.9	13.9
T10	14.1	15.2	16.2		14.7
T11	15.0	17.4	16.1		16.9
T12	14.7	15.8	15.9	15.0	16.5

the pedicle width of the thoracic spine to have a smaller diameter at the midthoracic region from T4 to T8-T9. Largest linear values are usually found at the ends of thoracic spine (T1-T2 and T11)[25,39,45,53,55,62] (Table 3–5).

Pedicle Height

All researchers measured the pedicle height in its shortest segment. The results did not demonstrate any significant difference between the studies. The values did not vary with respect to gender or right or left sides.[25,39,45,53,55,62] A height of 8.4 mm at T1 increased rapidly to 12.4 mm at T3. Between T3 and T8, the height averaged 10.1 mm to 11.9 mm. From T8 to T12, there was another linear increase of ~1 mm per vertebral level. The largest pedicle height was at T11 or T12.[39,45] In general the pedicle height appears to inconsistently increase in size from T1 to T10, T11, or T12[39,45,53,55,56,62] (Table 3–6).

Pedicle Transverse Angle

Panjabi et al[45] defined pedicle angles from a pedicle centerline with respect to the transverse plane. In all cadaveric studies the measurements of the pedicle angle were based on a Steinmann pin inserted into the cancellous portion of the pedicle with is relationship to the transverse plane.[25,39,53,55,62] There was a significant difference

between most of the reports. The reasons for this are most likely caused by differences in technique.

Panjabi et al[45] encountered a general left/right symmetry. The inclination with the transverse plane remained relatively constant from T3 to T11 at ~9 degrees. The angle jumped from 7.6 degrees at T1 to 17.9 degrees at T2, and from 8.7 degrees at T11 to 5.3 degrees at T12[45] (Table 3–7).

A general decreasing trend in the transverse pedicle angle from cephalad to caudal was found in all the others series with no significant difference in gender. The greatest angulation in the transverse plane was found at T1[25,39,53,55,62] (Table 3–7).

Pedicle Sagittal Angle

As in the transverse angle the sagittal measurements were performed from a pedicle centerline with respect to the sagittal plane. Cadaveric studies used a pin inserted into the cancellous portion of the pedicle in relation with an end-plate line.[45]

Panjabi et al[45] encountered a progression of inclination relative to the sagittal plane decreasing generally from ~27 degrees at T1 to 10 degrees at T12. The reports of Ebraheim et al[25] have related the major angulation at T6 for both male and females, at ~27 degrees. At T1 the angulation was 23.3 degrees, which remained relatively constant until T12 with a change to 20.4 degrees.[25] Zindrick et al[62] showed the minor angulation at T1 to be 12.6 degrees and T12 to be 11.6 degrees (Table 3–8).

Pedicle and Pedicle Axis Length

Avoidance of anterior cortex perforation is the goal of this measurement. Unwanted consequences due to important structures could occur secondary to perforation of the anterior vertebral body wall.[42] Relations between vertebrae and vital structures such as the aorta, the vena cava, the esophagus, and the lung are of importance to spine surgeons.

TABLE 3–7 Thoracic Anatomy: Pedicle Transverse Angle

	Vaccaro	Zindrick	McCormick	Scoles	Panjabi	Ebraheim
T1		26.6	14.1	29.8	7.6	39.4
T2		19.1	15.3		17.9	35.4
T3		14.6	10.0	15.3	9.4	27.1
T4	13.9	12.6	5.8		10.5	29.1
T5	12.6	9.4	7.2		7.6	24.3
T6	8.6	9.6	8.6	10.2	9.6	25.9
T7	7.4	8.7	8.6		12.1	24.8
T8	6.9	8.1	4.6		11.1	26.4
T9	7.1	7.6	4.0	9.2	8.5	21.1
T10	4.1	4.6	10.1		7.3	19.6
T11	0.7	1.2	6.5		8.7	21.5
T12	7.3	−4.2	3.7	9.5	5.3	15.4

TABLE 3–8 Thoracic Anatomy: Pedicle Sagittal Angle

	Zindrick	Panjabi	Ebraheim
T1	12.6	27.0	23.3
T2	17.5	28.9	23.4
T3	17.3	22.5	22.1
T4	16.3	21.8	23.1
T5	15.0	20.2	24.6
T6	15.0	19.4	27.3
T7	15.7	23.4	23.6
T8	16.6	22.5	20.4
T9	16.0	19.3	17.9
T10	16.8	14.4	17.5
T11	15.4	12.9	19.9
T12	11.6	10.0	20.4

Three excellent studies were selected to describe this anatomy, those of Zindrick, Scoles, and Vaccaro.[53,55,62] They used measurements in different specimens but used the same parameters. The distance between the anterior cortex of the vertebral body from the most posterior aspect of the lamina and facet (entry point to pedicle) along the pedicle axis were designated as the pedicle axis length.

Differences were seen between the studies. Scoles et al[53] had the smallest dimensions, except at T12. The longest length was at T12, 43 mm to 46.6 mm[53,55] (Table **3–9**).

Shortest distance of 3.20 mm was found at T1.[53] In general, the length of the pedicle increases gradually from T1 to T12 in all studies with the exception of the Zindrick et al[62] report, in which there is a slight decrease from T10 to T12. The reports have shown a significant difference between males and females. In the male population we see the greatest dimensions ranged 2 to 3 mm more than in females (Table **3–9**).

Some authors also related the real pedicle length as the distance from the posterior aspect of the lamina and facet to the posterior cortex of the vertebral body or posterior longitudinal ligament along the pedicle axis. In these reports the distance from T1 to T10 increases gradually, and then decrease slightly to T12 with no significant difference between genders. The smallest distance was found at T1 (9.6 mm) and the greatest at T10 (13.5 mm).[25,39]

TABLE 3–9 Thoracic Anatomy: Pedicle Length (mm)

	Vaccaro	Zindrick	Scoles
T1		36.9	32.0
T2		35.7	
T3		37.7	31.6
T4	44.1	38.5	
T5	39.3	41.9	
T6	38.9	42.1	37.7
T7	43.6	44.6	
T8	44.7	43.4	
T9	43.5	45.2	41.9
T10	44.1	44.0	
T11	40.8	41.8	
T12	46.6	38.6	43.3

Entry Point to the Thoracic Pedicle

Many authors used the midline of the transverse process and the facet as a reliable landmark for craniocaudal projection of the pedicle in the thoracic spine.[15,25,36,37,39,51]

Roy-Camille et al[51] suggested that the entry point for the pedicle in the thoracic spine lies at the junction between midlines of the facet joint and the transverse process. Magerl[37] recommended that the starting point in the lower thoracic pedicle be at the junction of the lateral margin of the facet and the midline of the transverse process. An et al[15] suggested that the entry point in the upper thoracic pedicle should be at the midportion of the transverse process and 1 mm below the facet joint. Louis[36] considered that different levels should have different entrances. Above T3, the point would be 3 mm below the inferior facet and 3 mm medial to the lateral margin of the facet. At T4 to T10, this point should be more medial to the lateral margin of the facet.[36] Hou et al[31] showed that this point, at the lower thoracic pedicle (T9-T12), is rostral to the transverse process midline at T9 and then approaches the transverse process descending the lumbar spine. Ebraheim et al[25] recorded that the correct entry point to the pedicle in their reports was 7 to 8 mm medial to the lateral edge of the superior facet and 3 to 4 mm superior to the transverse process midline for T1 and T2. For T3 to T12 this point was 4 to 5 mm medial to the lateral margin of the facet and 5 to 8 mm superior to the midline of the transverse process. McCormack et al[39] related that we can find the rostral-caudal distance of the transverse process to the pedicle axis by a simple equation: $D = 7.9 - [1.2 \times TL]$ where TL stands for the thoracic level. We can see from this equation that the transverse process midline is rostral to the pedicle in the upper thoracic spine and caudal to the pedicle in the lower thoracic spine. The crossover occurs at the T6-T7 region.[39]

■ Pars Interarticularis

Panjabi et al[45] reported that the pars interarticularis area gradually increases from T4 to T11. The area at T3 was ~90 mm^2, and at T11 was 160 mm^2, which then decreases suddenly at T12 to 98 mm^2 secondary to the inferior facets changing from the thoracic type to lumbar type.

■ Spinous Process

The spinous process arises from the center of the posterior arch and projects dorsally and caudally. This projection is the attachment for many muscles.[16,19,20,42,50,54]

The spinous process length was measured from the superior end plate line to the most inferoposterior tip. At T1 it was ~50 mm with no significant changes until T11. At this level it decreases to 46 mm, which it maintains to T12.[45]

■ Transverse Process

The transverse processes are situated at the junction of the laminae and pedicles and then extend laterally and dorsally. They terminate laterally at the costal facets, adding support to the ribs. They are also attachments for many muscles.[19,20,29,30,42,54]

The transverse process width was defined as the distance from the tip of the left transverse process to that of the right side.[45] A decrease was found from T1 to T4, remained constant to T10, and then decreases from T10 to T12. The largest distance found at T1 was 75 mm, and the shortest distance was at T12 with 46 mm.[45]

■ Costotransverse and Costovertebral Articulation

The thoracic vertebrae are distinguished by either a costotransverse or a costovertebral complex. Each vertebra has a costal process developing into the ribs. They are located on the ventrolateral region of the vertebral body and articulate with the vertebral bodies by costal facets. We can see also another articulation on the transverse process except at T11 and T12.[19,20,29,30,42,54]

■ Thoracic Articular Facets

The superior and inferior facets arise from the upper and lower part of the pedicle. The superior facet has its articular surface on the dorsal aspect and has a circular or semicircular shape, whereas the inferior facet has its orientation on the ventral aspect with a semilunar shape. In general the thoracic articular facets are oriented in a more coronal direction.[19,20,29,30,42,45,54]

Facet Width

Significant differences between male and female facet widths have been noted.[26,44] The largest superior facet width in men was found at T1 with 15.1 mm, whereas in women it was at T10 with 11.2 mm.[26] Panjabi et al[44] noted a gradual decrease from 13.3 mm at T1 to 9.6 mm at T7, and a slight increase from 10 mm at T8 to 11.2 mm at T12. The inferior facet width was reported to be between 11.9 mm and 11.4 mm in the thoracic spine.[26,44]

TABLE 3–10 Lumbar Anatomy: Body Height

	Panjabi	Scoles	Berry
L1	23.8	27.4	25.8
L2	24.3		25.2
L3	23.8	27.4	26.0
L4	24.1		26.4
L5	22.9	27.6	23.1

Facet Angles

Ebraheim et al[26] defined the facet angle as the angle between the midsagittal plane and the slope of the facets measured in the axial plane. A constant change at the superior facet angle was observed, ~76.6 to 81.1 degrees.

The largest inferior facet angle in both men and women was found at T12 and an increase was noted from T8 to T12. The measurements from T1 to T10 showed a constant and slight increase (75.2 to 79.9 degrees) with a marked change occurring from T10 (79.9 degrees) to T11 (87.6 degrees) and T12 (107.7 degrees).[26,44]

Lumbar Anatomy

The lumbar vertebrae are responsible for supporting the cervical and thoracic segments; therefore, they have the largest bony elements bodies of the vertebral column.

Lumbar Vertebral Body

The lumbar vertebral bodies are the largest in the spine. They have their greatest diameter in the transverse aspect. Their end-plate distances or body heights are deeper and thicker ventrally than dorsally.[18,20,43,53,54]

The vertebral body height, as measured by several authors, did not demonstrate a major difference between male and female specimens (Table 3–10). There was a slight increase in the body width from L1 to L5. At L5, the largest value ranged 49.4 mm to 52.9 mm (Table 3–11). Vertebral body depth or anteroposterior (AP) diameter was relatively constant in its values in all reports[18,35,43,55] (Table 3–12).

Lumbar Pedicle

The pedicle of the lumbar spine has been the target of numerous studies due to its prominence as a site of transpedicular and percutaneous spinal procedures to reach the vertebral body for fixation.[1–14,17,18,20,43,47–49,51–56,59–61]

TABLE 3–11 Lumbar Anatomy: Body Width

	Panjabi	Scoles	Berry
L1	43.3	44.3	49.1
L2	45.5		54.8
L3	48.0	48.4	53.8
L4	49.5		50.9
L5	49.4	52.9	52.7

TABLE 3–12 Lumbar Anatomy: Body Anteroposterior Diameter (mm)

	Panjabi	Scoles	Berry	Krag
L1	35.3	29.5	32.3	31.0
L2	34.9		33.4	32.5
L3	34.8	32.6	34.2	30.5
L4	33.9		35.6	32.0
L5	33.2	34.5	34.5	33.0

TABLE 3–14 Lumbar Anatomy: Pedicle Height (mm)

	Panjabi	Ebraheim	Zindrick	Scoles	Robertson
L1	15.9	14.1	15.4	15.3	18.6
L2	14.9	14.2	15.0		18.6
L3	14.4	13.9	14.9	14.1	18.6
L4	15.4	12.7	14.8		17.8
L5	19.6	11.4	14.0	16.2	17.6

Pedicle Width

Pedicle width is defined as the shortest linear dimension of the pedicle in the transverse plane.[24,41,43,53,60]

Olsewski et al[41] compared the results of direct cadaver measurements to radiographic studies and revealed a difference of almost 2 mm greater on the radiographic records.

As expected, the largest pedicle width was at L5 with a mean of 18 mm. The shortest pedicle dimension was at L1 with a mean value of 7.4 mm[24,41,43,60] (Table **3–13**).

Pedicle Height

Pedicle height was defined as the shortest linear dimension of the pedicle in the sagittal plane.[25,45,48,51,55,61]

Scoles et al[53] and Zindrick et al[62] showed a constancy in the dimensions from L1 to L5. Panjabi et al[45] reported values ranging from 15.9 mm at L1 to 19.6 mm at L5. Ebraheim et al[25] related a decrease in these dimensions from L1 to L5 (14.1 mm to 11.4 mm, respectively). Robertson and Stewart[49] described the largest pedicle height at L1 (18.6 mm) (Table **3–14**).

Pedicle Transverse Angle

The transverse angle was defined as an angle in the transverse plane measured between a line through the pedicle axis and a line parallel to the vertebral midline.[25,45,53,62]

Significant variation was found between several studies. This was probably due to measuring techniques and starting points used to measure the angulations. An increase from L1 to L5 was noted in all reports.

Panjabi et al showed results ranging from 14.5 degrees at L1 to 24.6 degrees at L5. Scoles et al reported values of 11.6 degrees at L1 and 23.1 degrees at L5. Ebraheim et al also related an increase from L1 (25.8 degrees) to L5 (40.6 degrees). Zindrick et al also found similar results[24,43,53,62] (Table **3–15**).

Pedicle Sagittal Angle

The sagittal angle was defined as an angle in the sagittal plane measured between a line through the pedicle axis and a line parallel to the superior end plate.[24,41,43,62]

An increase of ~2.6 degrees at L1 to 5.5 degrees at L5 was reported by Panjabi. Ebraheim showed a slight decrease from 6.7 degrees at L1 to 2.6 degrees at L5. Olsewski showed no significant difference in the sagittal angle of the pedicle between radiographic and cadaveric measurements. Their findings ranged from 6.2 degrees to 7.4 degrees[24,41,43] (Table **3–16**).

Pedicle Length

Pedicle length was defined as the distance from the posterior cortex of the lamina to the anterior aspect of the cortex of the vertebral body through the pedicle axis.[25,43,55,61] One anatomic study reported a significant difference between measurements of cadaver dissections compared with radiographic findings.[41] The radiographic measurements were consistently larger than the cadaver measurements, ranging from 2.5 to 5.2 mm.[41]

Several investigators reported L3 to have the longest pedicle, ranging from 50.1 mm to 52.8 mm.[25,55,61] In another study, L4 was noted to be the vertebra with the longest pedicle length, 55.3 mm.[43] The smallest pedicle length was found to be at L1[25,43,55,61] (Table **3–17**).

Interpedicular Distance

The interpedicular distance is the transverse diameter of the spinal canal measured between the medial aspect of both pedicles.[25,43,55]

The interpedicular distance increased from L1 to L5. The measurements ranged from 22.2 mm at L1 to 27.1 mm at L5[25,43,55] (Table **3–18**).

TABLE 3–13 Lumbar Anatomy: Pedicle Width

	Panjabi	Ebraheim	Zindrick	Scoles	Olsewski
L1	8.6	7.4	8.7	8.3	8.5
L2	8.3	8.4	8.9		8.6
L3	10.2	9.8	10.3	9.1	9.7
L4	14.1	12.8	12.9		12.7
L5	18.6	17.6	18.0	9.7	19.1

TABLE 3–15 Lumbar Anatomy: Pedicle Transverse Angle

	Panjabi	Ebraheim	Zindrick	Scoles
L1	14.5	25.8	10.9	11.6
L2	14.1	27.3	12.0	
L3	18.5	29.4	14.4	14.7
L4	16.0	33.6	17.7	
L5	24.6	40.6	29.8	23.1

TABLE 3–16 Lumbar Anatomy: Pedicle Sagittal Angle

	Panjabi	Ebraheim	Zindrick	Olsewski
L1	2.6	6.7	2.4	6.8
L2	2.7	5.1	1.8	6.2
L3	2.7	3.9	0.2	6.8
L4	3.9	3.6	0.2	7.4
L5	5.5	2.7	−1.8	7.4

TABLE 3–18 Lumbar Anatomy: Interpedicular Distance (mm)

	Scoles	Ebraheim	Panjabi
L1	22.2	23.5	23.7
L2		23.9	23.8
L3	22.8	24.1	24.3
L4		23.2	25.4
L5	25.9	24.4	27.1

Relations between Pedicle and Neural Structures

Pedicle–inferior nerve root distance, pedicle–superior nerve root distance, and pedicle–dural sac distance are important measurements for the surgeon performing either open or closed procedures.[17,28]

The mean distances from the pedicle to the dural sac ranged from ~1 mm at L1 to 2 mm at L5.[17,28]

The mean distances from the pedicle to the nerve roots superiorly ranged from 4.6 mm at L1 to 5.7 mm at L5 according to a study by Ebraheim et al.[28] Inferiorly the distance was 1.4 at L1 to 1.6 mm at L5.[28] Attar et al[17] reported a range of 2.9 mm to 6.2 mm superiorly and 0.8 mm to 2.8 mm inferiorly.

Projection of the Pedicle at the Posterior Aspect of the Vertebra

The lateral edge of the superior facet joint and the transverse process midline are usually reliable landmarks on the posterior aspect of the lumbar spine to reach the pedicle entry point.[25]

Roy-Camille et al described a starting point for screw insertion into the lumbar pedicle as a crossing of two lines on a bone crest. The horizontal line is the midtransverse process line and a midfacet line 1 mm under the facet joint gives the vertical line. Magerl[37] stated that a starting point for the pedicle entry should be the crossing of the lateral edge of the superior facet and the midtransverse line. Weinstein et al[60] suggested the lateral and inferior corner of the superior facet joint was a suitable pedicle entry point. Ebraheim et al[26] named the entry point the pedicle axis projection. The point is superior to the midtransverse line by 3.9 mm at L1, 2.75 mm at L2, and 1.3 mm at L3. This point was inferior to the midtransverse line by 0.5 mm at L4 and 1.4 mm at L5.[26]

TABLE 3–17 Lumbar Anatomy: Pedicle Length (mm)

	Panjabi	Ebraheim	Zindrick	Olsewski
L1	50.9	48.1	50.7	45.8
L2		48.7	51.9	49.2
L3	52.8	50.1	51.9	51.7
L4		49.2	49.7	55.3
L5	52.5	48.3	51.0	49.2

Spinous Process

The spinous process of the lumbar spine are not as prominent as those of the thoracic spine and they are directed more cranially.[19,20,22,44,45,51,55]

Panjabi's group[45] measured the spinous process from the center of the superior end plate to the most inferior tip. They found values ranging from 68 mm at L1 to 72 mm at L3. At L5 the value decreased again to 68 mm.

Transverse Process

These bony processes are located laterally to the pedicles and arise from the junction of the lamina and pedicle in the upper three lumbar vertebrae. At the fourth and fifth vertebrae these processes arise from the pedicle and the posterior parts of the vertebral bodies. They are shortest at the first lumbar vertebra. There is an increase in size at the third lumbar vertebra. The size then decreases at the second, fourth, and fifth processes.[20,22,45,51,55]

Lumbar Articular Facets

In the lumbar spine, the articular processes are different from the cervical and thoracic levels. One of the most important differences is the angle made with the sagittal plane. The facets of the lumbar vertebrae are oriented from 120 degrees to 150 degrees from the sagittal plane, whereas the cervical and thoracic vertebrae are from 60 degrees to 90 degrees from the same plane.[20,45,55,58,59] The inferior articular processes have a convex surface turned ventrally and laterally. The superior articular process is concave and its surface is directed dorsally and medially to embrace the inferior process cranially.[20,55]

The dimensions of the facets increase significantly in the lumbar region. No significant difference was found between the sides of the superior and inferior facet heights. A small difference was noted between the superior and inferior facets, whereas the inferior was somewhat larger than the superior facet for a mean value of 1.8 mm. At the superior facets the largest height was found at L5, 17.5 mm, and the shortest at L1, 12.2 mm. The inferior facet showed values ranging from 15.3 mm at L1 to 18.4 mm at L5. The facet width of both the

TABLE 3–19 Lumbar Anatomy

	Superior Articular Facet			
	Facet Height	*Facet Width*	*Transverse Angle*	*Sagittal Angle*
L1	12.2	10.5	82.9	139.1
L2	14.6	11.4	85.7	135.4
L3	15.9	13.9	81.9	131.5
L4	17.3	15.3	81.2	120.8
L5	17.5	14.9	86.0	117.6
	Inferior Articular Facet			
	Facet Height	*Facet Width*	*Transverse Angle*	*Sagittal Angle*
L1	15.7	10.7	81.4	152.1
L2	16.3	12.7	82.8	142.5
L3	16.4	13.4	75.6	130.6
L4	15.6	14.1	70.5	112.7
L5	17.3	16.1	71.0	127.6

superior and inferior facets have almost the same values[45] (Table **3–19**).

At the thoracolumbar junction there is a marked change in the sagittal angle of the facets. This change is noted at the inferior facet of T12 and at the superior facet of L1. The superior facet angle changed from almost 70 degrees at T12 to 137 degrees at L1. From L1 to L5 the angles decrease from 137 degrees at L1 to 118 degrees at L5[45] (Table **3–19**).

■ Conclusion

Numerous excellent studies have been presented to provide the physician and surgeon with spinal anatomic details. Each study had its own set of specific data concerning bony anatomy. Even though the studies may differ in certain angles, heights, lengths, and other measurements, the basic anatomy is the same. Students of anatomy will learn the details that are important to their practice. The anatomic spinal studies are only guidelines for each student. A good comprehension and understanding of spinal anatomy and an appreciation of the variations will aid the spine practitioner in reaching targeted bony structures. This chapter provides surgeons, radiologists, spine physicians, and others some insight into the bony landmarks of the thoracic and lumbar vertebrae, with the intention to achieve better results for any spine approach, open or closed.

REFERENCES

1. Jensen ME, Evans AJ, Mathis JM, Kallmes DF, Cloft HJ, Dion JE. Percutaneous polymethylmethacrylate vertebroplasty in the treatment of osteoporotic vertebral body compression fractures: technical aspects. AJNR Am J Neuroradiol 1997;18:1897–1904
2. Mathis JM, Barr JD, Belkoff SM, Barr MS, Jensen ME, Deramond H. Percutaneous vertebroplasty: a developing standard of care for vertebral compression fractures. AJNR Am J Neuroradiol 2001;22:373–381
3. Galibert P, Deramond H, Rosat P, Legars D. Note preliminaire sur le traitement desangiomes vertebraux par vertebroplastie percutanee. Neurochirurgie 1987;33:166–168
4. Deramond H, Depriester C, Toussaint P. Percutaneous vertebroplasty with polymethylmethacrylate: technique, indications, and results. Radiol Clin North Am 1998;36:533–546
5. Deramond H, Galibert R, Debussche-Depriester C. Percutaneous vertebroplasty with methylmethacrylate: technique, method, results. Radiology 1990;117(suppl):352
6. Debussche-Depriester C, Deramond H, Fardellone P, et al. Percutaneous vertebroplasty with acrylic cement in the treatment of osteoporotic vertebral crush fracture syndrome. Neuroradiology 1991;33:149–152
7. Gangi A, Kastler BA, Dietmann JL. Percutaneous vertebroplasty guided by a combination of CT and fluoroscopy. AJNR Am J Neuroradiol 1994;15:83–86
8. Barr JD, Barr MS, Lemley TJ, McCann RM. Percutaneous vertebroplasty for pain relief and spinal stabilization. Spine 2000;25:923–928
9. Cotton A, Boutry N, Cortet B, et al. Percutaneous vertebroplasty: state of the art. Radiographics 1998;18:311–323
10. O'Brien JP, Sims JT, Evans AJ. Vertebroplasty in patients with severe vertebral compression fractures: a technical report. AJNR Am J Neuroradiol 2000;21:1555–1558
11. Riggs BL, Melton LJ III. The worldwide problem of osteoporosis: insights afforded by the epidemiology. Bone 1995;17:505S–511S
12. Tohmel AG, Mathis JM, Fenton DC, Levine AM, Belkoff SM. Biomechanical efficacy of unipedicular versus bipedicular vertebroplasty for the management of osteoporotic compression fractures. Spine 1999;24:1772–1776
13. Weill A, Chiras C, Simon JM, et al. Spinal metastases: indications for and results of percutaneous injection of acrylic surgical cement. Radiology 1996;199:241–247
14. Stringham DR, Hadjipavlou A, Dzioba RB, Lander P. Percutaneous transpedicular biopsy of the spine. Spine 1994;19:1985–1991
15. An HS, Gordin R, Renner K. Anatomic considerations for plate-screw fixation of the cervical spine. Spine 1991;16(suppl):S548–S551
16. Arey LB. Developmental Anatomy, 5th ed. Philadelphia: WB Saunders, 1978:363–389
17. Attar A, Ugur HC, Uz A, Tekdemir I, Egemen N, Gency Y. Lumbar pedicle: surgical anatomic evaluation and relationships. Eur Spine J 2001;10(1):10–15
18. Berry JL, Moran JM, Berg WS, Steff AD. A morphometric study of human lumbar and selected thoracic vertebrae. Spine 1987;12:362–367

19. Breathnach AS. Frazer's Anatomy of Human Skeleton, 6th ed. Boston: Little, Brown, 1965

20. Clemente CD. Gray's Anatomy, 30th American ed. Baltimore: Williams & Wilkins, 1984:114–422

21. Crock HV. An Atlas of Vascular Anatomy of the Skeleton and Spinal Cord. St. Louis: Mosby, 1996

22. Dwyer AP. Clinically relevant anatomy. In: Wiesel SW, Weinstein JN, Herskowitz H, Dvorak J, Bell G, eds. The Lumbar Spine, 2nd ed, vol 1. Philadelphia: WB Saunders, 1996:57–73

23. Ebraheim NA, Jabaly G, Xu R, Yeasting RA. Anatomic relations of the thoracic pedicle to the adjacent neural structures. Spine 1997;22:1553–1557

24. Ebraheim N, Rollins JR, Xu R, Yeasting RA. Projection of the lumbar pedicle and its morphometric analysis. Spine 1996;21: 1296–1300

25. Ebraheim NA, Xu R, Ahmad M, Yeasting RA. Projection of the thoracic pedicle and its morphometric analysis. Spine 1997;22:233–238

26. Ebraheim NA, Xu R, Ahmad M, Yeasting RA. The quantitative anatomy of the thoracic facet and the posterior projection of its inferior facet. Spine 1997;22:1811–1818

27. Ebraheim N, Xu R, Darwich M, Yeasting RA. Anatomic relations between the lumbar pedicle and the adjacent neural structures. Spine 1997;22:2338–2341

28. Ebraheim NA, Xu R, Farouq A, Yeasting RA. The quantitative anatomy of the iliac vessels and their relation to anterior lumbosacral approach. J Spinal Disord 1996;9:414–417

29. Ferner H. Pernkopf Atlas of Topographical and Applied Human Anatomy. Baltimore: Urban & Schwarzenberg, 1980

30. Ferner H, Staubesand J. Sobotta Atlas of Human Anatomy. Baltimore: Urban & Schwarzenberg, 1983

31. Hou S, Hu R, Shi Y. Pedicle morphology of the lower thoracic and lumbar spine in a Chinese population. Spine 1993;18:1850–1855

32. Kim NH, Lee HM, Chung IH, Kim HJ, Kim SJ. Morphometric study of the pedicles of the thoracic and lumbar vertebrae in Koreans. Spine 1994;19:1390–1394

33. Kothe R, O'Holleran JD, Liv W, Panjabi MN. Internal architecture of the thoracic pedicle spine. Spine 1996;21:264–270

34. Krag MH, Weaver DL, Beynnon BD, Haugh LD. Morphometry of the thoracic and lumbar spine related to transpedicular screw placement for surgical spinal fixation. Spine 1988;13:27–32

35. Larsell O. The nervous system. In: Shaeffer JP. ed. Morris' Human Anatomy. Philadelphia: Blackstone, 1947:854–1177

36. Louis R. Spinal internal fixation with Louis instrumentation. In: An HS, Cotler JM, eds. Spinal Instrumentation. Baltimore: Williams & Wilkins, 1992:183–196

37. Magerl FP. Stabilization of the lower thoracic and lumbar spine with external skeletal fixation. Clin Orthop 1984;189:125–141

38. McBride AD, Parker LM. Anatomy and exploration. In: Regan JJ, McAfee PC, Mack MJ, eds. Atlas of Endoscopic Spine Surgery. St. Louis: Quality Medical Publishing, 1995:91–113

39. McCormack BM, Benzel EC, Adams MS, Baldwin NG, Rupp FW, Maher DJ. Anatomy of the thoracic pedicle. Neurosurgery 1995;37:303–308

40. Oda I, Abumik LUD, Shono Y, Kanada K. Biomechanical rule of the posterior elements, costovertebral joints, and rib cage in the stability of the thoracic spine. Spine 1996;21:1423–1429

41. Olsewski JM, Simmons EH, Kallen FC, Wendel F, Severin CM, Berens DL. Morphometric of the lumbar spine: anatomic perspectives related to transpedicular fixation. J Bone Joint Surg Am 1990;72: 541–549

42. Pait TG, Türe U, Arnautovic KI, Tribell RM. Surgical anatomy of the thoracic spine. In: Dickman CA, Rosenthal D, Perin N, eds. Thoracoscopic Spine Surgery. New York: Thieme Medical, 1998:57–67

43. Panjabi MM, Goel V, Oxland T, Duranceau J, Krag M, Price M. Human lumbar vertebra: quantitative three-dimensional anatomy. Spine 1992;17:299–306

44. Panjabi MM, Oxland T, Tarata K, Goel V, Duranceau J, Krag M. Articular facets of the human spine: quantitative three-dimensional anatomy. Spine 1993;18:1298–1310

45. Panjabi MM, Tarata K, Goel V, et al. Thoracic human vertebrae: quantitative three-dimensional anatomy. Spine 1991;16:888–901

46. Platzer W. Pernkopf Anatomie. Munich: Urban & Schwarzenberg, 1987

47. Postacchini F, Ripani M, Carpano S. Morphometry of the lumbar vertebrae: an anatomic study in two Caucasoid ethnic groups. Clin Orthop 1983;172:296–303

48. Robertson PA, Novotny JE, Grobler LJ, Agbai JU. Reliability of axial landmarks for pedicle screw placement in the lower lumbar spine. Spine 1998;23:60–66

49. Robertson PA, Stewart NR. The radiologic anatomy of the lumbar and lumbosacral pedicles. Spine 2000;25:709–715

50. Romanes GJ. Cunningham's Textbook of Anatomy, 12th ed. Oxford: Oxford University Press, 1981:220–227

51. Roy-Camille R, Mazel C, Laville C. Roy-Camille posterior screw plate fixation for cervical, thoracic, lumbar spine and sacrum. In: An HS, Cotler JM, eds. Spinal Instrumentation. Baltimore: Williams and Wilkins, 1992:167–181

52. Roy-Camille R, Saillant G, Mazel C. Internal fixation of the lumbar spine with pedicle screw plating. Clin Orthop 1986;203:7–17

53. Scoles PV, Linton AE, Latimer B, Levy ME, Digiovanni BF. Vertebral body and posterior element morphology: the normal spine in middle life. Spine 1998;13:1082–1086

54. Terry RJ. Osteology. In: Morris' Human Anatomy. Philadelphia: Blackstone, 1947:77–265

55. Vaccaro AR, Rizzolo SJ, Allardyce TJ, et al. Placement of pedicle screws in the thoracic spine. J Bone Joint Surg Am 1995;77: 1193–1199

56. Vaccaro AR, Rizzolo SJ, Balderston RA, et al. Placement of pedicle screws in the thoracic spine, II: An anatomical and radiographic assessment. J Bone Joint Surg Am 1995;77:1200–1205

57. Van Schaik JP. Lumbar facet joint morphology. J Spinal Disord 2000;13:88–89

58. Van Schaik JP, Verbies H, Van Schaik FD. The orientation of laminae and facet joints in the lower lumbar spine. Spine 1985; 10:59–63

59. Williams PL, Bannister LH, Berry MM, et al. Gray's Anatomy. London: Churchill Livingstone, 1995:522–543

60. Weinstein JN, Rydevik BL, Raushining W. Anatomic and technical considerations of pedicle screw fixation. Clin Orthop 1992;284: 34–46

61. White AA III, Panjabi MM. The problem of clinical instability in the human spine: a systemic approach. In: White AA III, Panjabi MM, eds. Clinical Biomechanics of the Spine. Philadelphia: J Lippincott, 1978:236–251

62. Zindrick MR, Wiltse LL, Doornik A, et al. Analysis of the morphometric characteristics of the thoracic and lumbar pedicles. Spine 1987;12:160–166

4

Outcome Measures for Vertebroplasty and Kyphoplasty

PETER C. GERSZTEN AND WILLIAM C. WELCH

Objectives: On completion of this chapter, the reader should be able to discuss (1) the characteristics of outcomes instruments and (2) the applicability to patients treated with vertebroplasty or kyphoplasty.

Accreditation: The American Association of Neurological Surgeons is accredited by the Accreditation Council for Continuing Medical Education to sponsor continuing medical education for physicians.

Credit: The American Association of Neurological Surgeons designates this continuing medical education activity for a maximum of 15 credits in Category I of the Physician's Recognition Award of the American Medical Association.

The Home Study Examination is online at www.aans.org/education/books/vertebro.asp

Outcomes research may be defined as the research on the management of patients that asks what treatment is effective and for whom in more realistic settings than the ones used in randomized, controlled trials. The emphasis of the study techniques is on an array of outcomes beyond simple restoration of normal and anatomic relationships and particularly on end points emphasizing the patient's assessment of pain, function, quality of life, and satisfaction with the results of the intervention. Table 4–1 lists outcomes measures relevant to orthopedic surgery and neurosurgery.[1] This chapter reviews the procedures of vertebroplasty and kyphoplasty with regard to outcomes measures and outcomes research.

■ Introduction to Outcomes Measures

Outcomes are measured both directly and indirectly, over differing periods of time, and with varying degrees of objectivity, reliability, and validity. Important *characteristics* of outcomes include the following: dimension of health (e.g., physiologic, physical, or emotional); directly observable phenomenon (alleviation of pain); timing (e.g., immediate response to medications, or results of a surgical procedure after 1 year); and directness of the relationship of outcome to processes of care.[2] Elements of the *measurement* of outcomes include

purpose, source of information, mode of data collection, and the agent responsible for analysis and interpretation. General considerations in outcomes evaluations include the following: (1) The end points should measure impairment or disability. (2) The determination of the outcome should include both the benefits and the risks of the procedure. (3) The outcome and complications should be documented according to a protocol. (4) The techniques used should be tested for their reliability, validity, and sensitivity. (5) When multiple end points are determined, statistical corrections should be used to examine these end points. (6) There should be a sufficient number of subjects.[3]

The criteria for choosing among available measures of medical outcomes are the reliability and validity of the instrument in the context of the specific disease process being examined. Methods of measurement must also be evaluated for their ability to yield observable differences within a reasonable time. Because of time involved with the cost of data collection, the development of brief measures of functional status and well-being are essential for their use in routine practice settings.[4]

If heterogeneous patient groups are included in longitudinal observational studies, some sort of measurement of the "case mix" is crucial for the proper interpretation of the effectiveness of the intervention.[5] The case mix refers to the features that increase the risk of a bad

TABLE 4–1 Examples of Outcome Measures in Neurosurgery[22]

Category	Examples
Physiologic	Range of motion
Anatomic	Tumor residual on imaging, solid fusion mass
Complications	Dural tear, infection
Physical examination	Neurologic deficits, ability to walk
Mortality	Length of survival
Health-related quality-of-life symptoms	Pain duration, severity, and frequency; diplopia
Functional status	Activities of daily living, physiologic functioning, social functioning
Role function	Employment status, disability compensation
Health care use and costs	Tests ordered, compensation, assistive devices required, medical care costs
Satisfaction	With treatment, with results; were expectations met?

TABLE 4–2 Factors to Consider in Selecting Outcome Measures[6]

Sensibility
Face and content validity for intended purpose: includes relevant items, excludes irrelevant items
Suited to study purpose: individual patient versus groups of patients; quality assessment versus clinical efficacy versus policy
Appropriate for patient population: children, adults, aged; English-speaking/non–English-speaking; sciatica versus low back pain versus malignancy
Setting: primary care versus specialty care; inpatient versus outpatient; urban versus rural; telephone versus written
Feasibility
Easy for patients to understand
Easy to use: appropriate length; self-administered versus interviewer; require special equipment or training?
Cost to administer, score, computerize, analyze
Results interpretable, easy to present
Reliability
Internal consistency
Interrater reliability
Intrarater reliability
Validity
Correlation with other outcome measures
Prediction of future events
Responsiveness
Able to detect subtle but clinically relevant change?

outcome or influence the choice of treatment. The purpose of a "case-mix adjustment" is to separate the effects of the treatment given from those of the preexisting health status of the patient and other factors such as age and socioeconomic status that may affect outcome measures. For example, the percentage of patients receiving workers' compensation benefits is frequently reported in series describing the outcome of spinal fusion surgery, as the presence of a compensable disability claim is known to influence the rate of favorable outcome.

The concepts of "efficacy" and "effectiveness" are important to the definition of outcomes. Efficacy reflects the level of benefit expected when health care services are applied under "ideal" conditions of use. In contrast, effectiveness concerns the level of benefit when services are rendered under ordinary circumstances by average practitioners for typical patients.[2] Efficacy indicates the outcomes that can ultimately be achieved with a given health care service and effectiveness reveals the outcomes that are presently reached. Differences between the two may provide insights into how improvements in health care delivery might be made by outcomes research.

There are several factors to consider in selecting the appropriate outcome measure. Table **4–2** shows some of the factors to consider in selecting outcomes measures. The most important criterion is choosing an outcome measure that is clinically sensible.[6] This means that it meets a clinician's judgment that the questionnaire is measuring what an investigator wants to measure and that the items represent the domain of interest in a reasonably comprehensive manner. The user must judge whether a given questionnaire is appropriate for his or her patient population and clinical setting. The feasibility of the questionnaire is another key feature. Will it be understandable in the given patient population? The

reliability and validity, as previously mentioned, are important to consider. The responsiveness of the outcome measure (Can it detect small but clinically important changes or differences?) must be documented. There are several statistical methods for quantifying these characteristics of a questionnaire that may be found in the literature.[6,7]

Finally, when selecting an outcome measure, it must be considered whether a proposed questionnaire can measure changes or differences at the level of disease severity likely to be observed. For example, a questionnaire that is designed to measure gross activities of daily living among hospitalized inpatients on a rehabilitation ward would be inappropriate for mildly ill patients with a backache in a primary care setting. Similarly, a questionnaire designed for use in general populations might be unable to register the severe dysfunction in highly specialized or inpatient settings.[6]

■ Specific Outcome Measures for Vertebroplasty and Kyphoplasty

Table **4–3** shows selected examples of specific questionnaires that have been used to measure health-related quality-of-life issues in patients with low back pain. The disease-specific functional measures are focused clearly on back-related problems, and therefore have obvious relevance both to patients and physicians. The instruments may be more responsive to back treatments than

TABLE 4–3 Selected Instruments for Measuring Aspects of Health-Related Quality of Life in Patients with Low Back Pain[6]

Category	Instrument	No. of Items	Approx. Time to Complete	Dimensions
Symptoms	McGill Pain Questionnaire[23]	26	15 minutes	Pain severity, affective response
	Visual Analog Scales	Variable	1 minute	Pain severity, frequency
	Chronic Pain Grade (VonKorff)	7	5 minutes	Pain intensity, perceived impact
	NASS* Questionnaire	12	3 minutes (for pain) (questions only)	Back pain, leg pain, numbness, weakness; frequency, severity, duration
	Dallas Pain Score[24]	16	5 minutes	Daily activities, work and leisure, anxiety-depression, social interest
Disease-specific functional status	Roland-Morris Disability Scale[25]	24	5 minutes	Various daily functions
	Oswestry Disability Questionnaire[20]	10	5 minutes	Self-care, lifting, walking, standing, sleeping, social, others
	Million instrument[26]	15	10 minutes	Various daily functions
	NASS* questionnaire	9	5 minutes	Adapted from Oswestry
Generic functional status	SF-36[27,28]	36	10 minutes	Physical function, role function, pain, vitality, mental health, health perception
	Sickness Impact Profile[29,30]	136	20 minutes	Ambulation, self care, emotional function, social function, household activities, work, recreation, sleep, others
	Nottingham Health Profile[31]	38	5 minutes	Physical mobility, pain, sleep, energy, social, emotional
	Duke Health Profile[32]	17	5 minutes	Social, psychological, physical
Role function	Health interview	3	1 minute	Days work absenteeism, days in bed, days limited activity
	Survey items[33] NASS* questionnaire	9	5 minutes	Work status, compensation status, job description

*The NASS questionnaire includes items related to symptoms (see also generic functional status measures), functional status, and role function, as well as medical history, comorbidity, and satisfaction.

generic instruments, and may accomplish this with fewer questions. On the other hand, the generic functional status questionnaires may help to identify complications or side effects in areas of function or organ systems that are not specifically spine related. Furthermore, they permit comparisons with a common metric between the impact of treating back problems and the impact of treating other medical conditions. For many research purposes, it may be optimal to include both disease-specific and generic functional status measures.[6]

There are several problems to consider when applying outcomes research to the evaluation of the procedures of vertebroplasty and kyphoplasty. To begin with, there are different opinions for the indications for the procedure. In addition, some claim that one technique is superior over the other. Furthermore there is no single nonsurgical therapy for direct comparison. There are also widely different opinions as to what signifies a successful outcome. Finally, there are multiple variations in techniques used. All of these factors complicate the application of outcomes measures to the study of both vertebroplasty and kyphoplasty.

To complicate matters further, there are multiple problems with the outcomes measures themselves. Often, there is a general lack of sensitivity for what is trying to be measured. In addition, there is a lack of responsiveness of

instruments to what the individual investigator is trying to measure. Often, these self-reported outcomes measures are long, and patients do not like to fill them out. Finally, there are limitations of disease-specific outcomes instruments. Normative scores may not be available and validation of the instrument may be lacking.

After overcoming the difficulty with outcomes instruments themselves, there are a variety of other problems with applying outcomes research to the study of vertebroplasty and kyphoplasty. Obtaining the data is difficult and cumbersome. The cost is quite high. Few individual researchers have the resources available to them to obtain these data, necessitating corporate sponsorship and funding of clinical trials. In addition, there are complicating factors specific to this patient population. These patients are often old and disabled and have a multitude of other medical comorbidities that confound the treatment.

There is currently no general consensus on the ideal follow-up necessary for this patient population. It is often the case that patients receive almost immediate relief in their pain symptoms following the procedures. If one were to follow them longer, it is quite likely that the occurrence of compression fractures at other levels resulting in recurrent pain would confound the initial successful results of the procedures. On the other hand, few critics would accept 48 hours as an adequate follow-up period. Other confounding issues include the fact that there is lack of uniformity of postprocedure and postoperative analgesics. Many patients might quickly be referred to a formal pain clinic with good results from oral analgesics. The use or nonuse of aggressive physical therapy is another potentially confounding factor.

A final factor to consider related to the applications of outcomes research to vertebroplasty and kyphoplasty is the problem of study bias. Can all patients who undergo a particular procedure by a particular provider be entered into a study? Some patients may be unwilling to participate in the study. Others may not be able to participate in proper follow-up evaluation because of health-related issues, geographic distance, or inconvenience. The question of whether or not the remaining study population is a representative sample of the overall patient population becomes relevant. Finally, the patient population treated by one researcher may or may not be similar to that of other practices. Such bias prevents other practitioners from accepting the results of the outcomes reported by a single physician.

■ Literature Review and Outcomes Measures

A review of the literature regarding the procedures of vertebroplasty and kyphoplasty reveals several small or moderate-sized series of treated patients. No large series evaluating the durability of vertebroplasty have been published to date.[8] In addition, no prospective, randomized trials comparing vertebroplasty with nonoperative medical therapy have been reported.[9] Rather than critically review the literature regarding these procedures, we review here the clinical studies that have been published and how they have utilized outcomes measures as part of their results. Table 4–4 lists selected studies and the outcomes measures that were used.

Because kyphoplasty has been performed in only the last 2 years, long-term data have not yet been reported in peer-reviewed journals.[9] Over 1500 fractures have been treated by kyphoplasty performed by investigators who are obliged to contribute their data. They report a 90 to 95% significant pain relief in patients treated with this procedure. Assessment of results and complications is not dependent on isolated literature reports as is the case with vertebroplasty. The ability to control the use to a limited number of investigators who must perform to high standards of reporting results and complications is an advantage of the manufacturer-supported study group approach to the investigation of this new technology.[9] Long-term outcomes, at the time of this publication, are simply not available for review. This section does not directly address or compare vertebroplasty with kyphoplasty.

Table 4–4 lists selected studies that have been published on vertebroplasty and kyphoplasty with information regarding the outcomes instruments utilized. It is apparent that the mean length of follow-up for the majority of these studies is rather short. The number of patients for these clinical studies is also relatively small. Finally, and most importantly, few of these studies have incorporated any form of outcomes instrument to measure the results of the procedure.

Barr et al[10] reported a retrospective review of 47 patients treated over a 4-year period. Vertebroplasty was used to treat both osteoporotic compression fractures as well as spinal column neoplasms. The clinical response utilized for the procedure was a verbal response by the patient to a pain scale. The follow-up ranged from 2 to 42 months with a mean of 18 months. No outcomes instruments were utilized in this study. Cortet et al[11] reported a prospective study of 16 patients. Vertebroplasty was performed for osteoporosis only in this cohort. The clinical responses utilized include the amount of analgesics taken by the patients as well as a variety of generic health status instruments. These outcomes instruments included a visual analog scale, the McGill-Melzak scoring

TABLE 4–4 Selected Studies on Vertebroplasty and Kyphoplasty with Outcomes Instruments Utilized

Reference	No. of Patients	Clinical Response Utilized	Outcomes Instruments Utilized	Length of Follow-Up
Barr et al, 2000	47	Verbal response to pain scale	None	mean <18 months
Cortet et al, 1999	16	Analgesic effect, generic health status instrument	Visual analog scale, McGill-Melzack scoring system, Nottingham Health Profile	6 months
Cyteval et al, 1999	20	Analgesic effect	Visual analog scale	6 months
Deramond et al, 1998	80	Verbal response to pain scale	None	1 months to 10 years.
Do et al, 1999	6	Radiographic response	None	<24 hours
Jensen et al, 1997	29	Verbal response to pain scale	None	<24 hours
Lieberman et al, 2001	30	Radiographic response	SF-36	3 months
Weill et al, 1996	37	Analgesic effect	None	7 mos.
Wong et al, 2000	85	Radiographic response; verbal response to pain scale	None	5 months

system, and the Noddingham Health Profile. The length of follow-up for this study was 6 months. Although a relatively small number of patients were included in this study, this was the only study that incorporated a variety of outcomes instruments. Cyteval et al[12] reported on a series of 20 patients who were treated with vertebroplasty for osteoporotic compression fractures. Clinical response was determined using analgesic effect. The outcomes instrument utilized was a visual analog scale. The length of follow-up was 6 months. No disease-specific outcomes instruments or generic health status instruments were utilized. Deramond et al[13] reported the largest series of 80 patients who were treated with vertebroplasty for a variety of indications over a 10-year period. The follow-up ranged from 1 month to 10 years. Immediate results were excellent in more than 90% of these cases, with complete relief of symptoms in patients capable of standing up and walking 24 hours after the procedure. Unfortunately, the clinical response used was a verbal response to a pain scale. No outcomes instruments were utilized. Do et al[14] reported on a subset of six patients out of a retrospective chart review of a series of 95 patients who were treated using vertebroplasty. These six patients all carried a diagnosis of vertebral osteonecrosis. The clinical response utilized was radiographic response. No outcomes instruments were utilized. The follow-up was less than 24 hours. The next reference is from Jensen et al[15,16] from the same clinical group. This study reported on 29 patients who were treated over a 3-year period. Once again, a follow-up of less than 24 hours was used. The clinical response utilized was a verbal response to a pain scale. No outcomes instruments were used. No long-term follow-up was obtained. The authors state in this paper that the long-term outcome in this patient population is currently being analyzed and will be the subject of a future publication.

Lieberman et al[17] most recently reported on 70 consecutive kyphoplasty procedures performed in 30 patients. The length of follow-up was 3 months. The clinical response utilized was a radiographic response. However, in this study, the medical outcome study (MOS) 36-Item Short Form Health Survey (SF-36) was utilized as the outcomes instrument. This study showed that the SF-36 scores for bodily pain and physical function were among those that showed significant improvement. Weill et al[18] reported on 37 patients who underwent vertebroplasty for both analgesia as well as stabilization of the vertebral column. The mean follow-up was 7 months. The main clinical response was analgesic event effect. Clear improvement was defined as enough of a decrease in the pain that the dose of analgesics could be reduced by at least 50% so that a nonnarcotic instead of a narcotic drug could be administered. No outcomes instruments were utilized. Finally, Wong et al[19] reported a series of 85 patients undergoing kyphoplasty. Clinical response was determined by radiographic response as well as a verbal response to a pain scale. The average follow-up was 5 months. Ninety-four percent of patients reported good or excellent pain relief. No other kyphoplasty clinical series results are referenced in this report.

■ Recommendations for Future Studies

To date, no prospective trials evaluating either vertebroplasty or kyphoplasty with noninvasive medical therapy have been reported. Data are currently being collected to evaluate these two techniques at several centers. One factor that has contributed to the problem of follow-up has been that this procedure is often performed by interventional radiologists. The patients are referred to the interventional radiologists by a wide variety of specialists including primary care physicians, neurosurgeons, orthopedic surgeons, oncologists, and rheumatologists. In most cases, the radiologists do not have access to patient follow-up information.

Not only is it essential to collect good and careful follow-up data on these patients, it is also necessary to apply well-described and accepted outcomes research techniques to the rigorous evaluation of these two treatments. This is not to say that these two treatments are not effective. The conclusion here is that the effectiveness of these techniques has not been adequately assessed using the latest in outcomes research methodologies. Future studies should include well-described and widely used outcomes instruments for low back pain in addition to general quality-of-life instruments. Disease-specific outcomes questionnaires, such as the Oswestry Low Back Pain Questionnaire[20] and the North American Spine Society Low Back Pain Questionnaire,[21] should be employed. In addition, pain scales such as visual analog scales should be widely utilized. Finally, health-related quality of life global outcomes scales should be incorporated into any future studies. Scales such as the SF-36 should at the very least be incorporated. These scales are well validated and easily accessible to all researchers; they are also quite easy to administer to patients.

It is unreasonable to expect that a randomized study will be successfully completed in which patients are randomized to either vertebroplasty or kyphoplasty versus no intervention. Although a general consensus has not been reached on the efficacy of these interventions, it is doubtful that patients would willingly enter into such a study, making accrual almost impossible.

From the review of a select group of studies that have been performed on both kyphoplasty and vertebroplasty, it appears that the immediate relief of pain in all patients regardless of the procedure is exceedingly high. It is the long-term effect of the procedure regarding improvement of pain and subsequent kyphosis that is in question. The calculation of a sample size necessary to determine an improvement of one procedure over another in the long-term depends on the expected long-term improvement. One way to approach this is as follows. One may hypothesize that approximately one third of patients will improve with noninterventional therapy (the natural history) and 75% will improve with either vertebroplasty or kyphoplasty. An "improvement" compared with the natural history may be conservatively defined as a 50% improvement in symptoms based on the results of the outcomes instruments utilized. Power calculations indicate that ~50 patients evenly randomized between a treatment and control group would be necessary to have at least an 80% chance (power = 0.80) of demonstrating this degree of improvement with a 95% significance level ($p > 0.05$).

Aside from a randomized trial comparing these interventions to noninvasive treatments for osteoporotic compression fractures, longitudinal cohort studies could provide a significant amount of important outcomes information. Length of follow-up would have to be at least 1 year and preferably 2 years, given the natural history of this disease process. A disease-specific outcomes instrument such as the Oswestry Low Back Pain Questionnaire would be most suitable. In addition, the SF-36 would be used. Studies have shown the sensitivity of the Bodily Pain section of the SF-36 is appropriate for patients treated with kyphoplasty.[17] A visual analog scale should also accompany the patient follow-up. The combination of these three outcomes instruments is fairly routine and easily obtained from patients. These instruments should be obtained immediately prior to intervention. A visual analog scale measurement would be applied immediately after treatment. A 2-year follow-up with interval assessments at 6 weeks, 3 months, 6 months, and 1 year would be ideal. If such prospectively obtained information were available for both kyphoplasty and vertebroplasty patients separately, then the outcomes could be directly compared without the need for a direct randomized study. These longitudinal cohort studies could also be designed to enroll case-controlled age-matched individuals. Such a case-controlled study would allow for the calculation of an odds ratio of improvement following intervention. Therefore, through careful study design, the need for an expensive, difficult, and in some sense unethical randomized clinical trial is not necessarily required for the generation of high-quality outcomes data. It is the responsibility of those who propose and perform these procedures to provide such data.

REFERENCES

1. Liang MH, Andersson G, Bombardier C, et al. Strategies for outcome research in spinal disorders: an introduction. Spine 1994;19(suppl 18):2037s–2040s

2. Lohr K. Outcome measurement: concepts and questions. Inquiry 1988;25:37–50

3. Keller RB, Rudicel SA, Liang MH. Outcomes research in orthopaedics. Instr Course Lect 1994;43:599–611

4. Steward AL, Hays RD, Ware JE Jr. The MOS short form general health survey: reliability and validity in a patient population. Med Care 1988;26:724–735

5. Greenfield S. The state of outcome research: are we on target? N Engl J Med 1989;320:1142–1143

6. Deyo RA, Andersson G, Bombardier C, et al. Outcome measures for studying patients with low back pain. Spine 1994;19(suppl 18):2032S–2036S

7. Guyatt G, Walter S, Norman G. Measuring change over time: assessing usefulness of evaluative instruments. J Chronic Dis 1987;40:171–178

8. Jensen M. Percutaneous vertebroplasty: a new therapy for the treatment of painful vertebral body compression fractures. Appl Radiol 2000:7–11

9. Mathis JM, Barr JD, Belkoff SM, Barr MS, Jensen ME, Deramond H. Percutaneous vertebroplasty: a developing standard of care for vertebral compression fractures. AJNR Am J Neuroradiol 2001; 22:373–381

10. Barr JD, Barr MS, Lemley TJ, McCann RM. Percutaneous vertebroplasty for pain relief and spinal stabilization. Spine 2000;25:923–928

11. Cortet B, Cotten A, Boutry N, et al. Percutaneous vertebroplasty in the treatment of osteoporotic vertebral compression fractures: an open prospective study. J Rheumatol 1999;26:2222–2228

12. Cyteval C, Sarrabere MP, Roux JO, et al. Acute osteoporotic vertebral collapse: open study on percutaneous injection of acrylic surgical cement in 20 patients. AJR 1999;173:1685–1690

13. Deramond H, Depriester C, Galibert P, Le Gars D. Percutaneous vertebroplasty with polymethylmethacrylate: technique, indications, and results. Radiol Clin North Am 1998;36:533–546

14. Do HM. Jensen ME, Marx WF, et al. Percutaneous vertebroplasty in vertebral osteonecrosis (Kummell's spondylitis). Neurosurg Focus 1999;1(Article 2)

15. Jensen ME, Evans AJ, Mathis JM, Kallmes DF, Cloft HJ, Dion JE. Percutaneous polymethylmethacrylate vertebroplasty in the treatment of osteoporotic vertebral body compression fractures: technical aspects. AJNR Am J Neurorad 1997;18:1897–1904

16. Jensen ME, Garfin SR, Fardon D. Vertebroplasty vs kyphoplasty. SpineLine 2001;11–14

17. Lieberman IH, Dudeney S, Reinhardt MK, Bell G. Initial outcome and efficacy of "kyphoplasty" in the treatment of painful osteoporotic vertebral compression fractures. Spine 2001;26:1631–1638

18. Weill A, Chiras J, Simon JM, Rose M, Sola-Martinez T, Enkaoua E. Spinal metastases: indications for and results of percutaneous injection of acrylic surgical cement. Radiology 1996;199:241–247

19. Wong W, RMA, Garfin S. Vertebroplasty/kyphoplasty. J Women's Imag 2000;2(3):117–124

20. Fairbank JC, Couper J, Davies JB, O'Brien JP. The Oswestry Low Back Pain Disability Questionnaire. Physiotherapy 1980;66: 271–273

21. Daltroy LH, Cats-Baril WL, Katz JN, Fossel AH, Liang MH. The North American Spine Society lumbar spine assessment instrument. Spine 1996;21:741–749

22. Gerszten PC. Outcomes research: a review. Neurosurgery 1998;43: 1146–1156

23. Melzack R. The McGill Pain Questionnaire: major properties and scoring methods. Pain 1975;1:277–299

24. Lawlis GF, Cuencas R, Selby D, McCoy CE. The development of the Dallas Pain Questionnaire: an assessment of the impact of spinal pain on behavior. Spine 1989;14:511–516

25. Roland M, Morris R. A study of the natural history of back pain, I: Development of a reliable and sensitive measure of disability in low-back pain. Spine 1983;8:141–144

26. Million R, Hall W, Nilsen KH, Baker RD, Jayson MI. Assessment of the progress of the back-pain patient. 1981 Volvo Award in Clinical Science. Spine 1982;7:204–212

27. McHorney CA, Ware JE Jr, Raczek AE. The MOS 36-Item Short Form Health Survey (SF-36), II: Psychometric and clinical tests of validity in measuring physician and mental health constructs. Med Care 1993;31:247–263

28. Ware JJ, Sherbourne CD. The MOS 36-Item Short-Form Health Survey (SF-36), I: Conceptual framework and item slection. Med Care 1992;30:473–483

29. Bergner M, Bobbitt RA, Carter WB, Gilson BS. The Sickness Impact Profile: development and final revision of a health status measure. Med Care 1981;19:787–805

30. Deyo RA, Diehl AK. Measuring physical and psychosocial function in patients with low-back pain. Spine 1983;8:635–642

31. Kind P. Carr-Hill R. The Nottingham Health Profile: a useful tool for epidemiologists? Soc Sci Med 1987;25:905–910

32. Parkerson GR, Broadhead WE, Tse CKJ. The Duke Health Profile: a 17-item measure of health and dysfunction. Med Care 1990;28: 1056–1069

33. Turczyn KM, Drury TF. An inventory of pain data from the National Center for Health Statistics, Vital and Health Statistics Series 1, No. 26. DHHS Publication No. (PHS) 92–1308. Washington, DC: DHHS, 1992

5

Techniques for Percutaneous Vertebroplasty

TORO KOIZUMI, R. V. CHAVALI, AND I. S. CHOI

Objectives: On completion of this chapter, the reader should be able to (1) discuss the technique of vertebroplasty and (2) identify potential complications.

Accreditation: The American Association of Neurological Surgeons is accredited by the Accreditation Council for Continuing Medical Education to sponsor continuing medical education for physicians.

Credit: The American Association of Neurological Surgeons designates this continuing medical education activity for a maximum of 15 credits in Category I of the Physician's Recognition Award of the American Medical Association.

The Home Study Examination is online at www.aans.org/education/books/vertebro.asp

Percutaneous vertebroplasty is a therapeutic procedure that involves injection of bone cement (polymethylmethacrylate, PMMA) into a cervical, thoracic, or lumbar vertebral body. The procedure is a minimally invasive procedure developed in Europe, being first described in France in 1987.[1] Percutaneous vertebroplasty has become an established technique for treatment of painful, osteoporotic compression fractures.[2–9] This procedure can be performed with excellent clinical results and a low complication rate. Over the past 4 years, we have treated over 250 patients suffering painful thoracic or lumbar compression fractures with percutaneous vertebroplasty. We describe our approach, technique, and clinical results for percutaneous vertebroplasty after having now treated more than 600 fractures.

■ Patient Selection

Patients with subacute or chronic fractures, and with focal pain attributable to the fracture are considered appropriate candidates. Care is taken to exclude those with pain related to other complicated spinal problems, such as primary disk herniation or spinal canal stenosis, or radicular pain from degenerative foraminal stenosis or facet arthropathy. Acute burst fractures with neurocompressive effects are considered a major contraindication to percutaneous vertebroplasty because of the risk for retropulsion of bone

and further neural compromise. We do, however, accept on occasion an acute compression fracture in patients who have been admitted for pain control without any of the above complicating factors if there is good imaging available, and those who suffer a compression fracture immediately following an improved period after a vertebroplasty.

We evaluate all outpatients in a multidisciplinary forum with an endocrinologist and orthopedic surgeon with spinal expertise. Inpatients are often consulted on individually, but we make every effort to have all team members aware of the patient's status.

The risks of the procedure, including bleeding, infection, allergic reaction, rib fractures,[8] errant placement of cement leading to potential pulmonary embolism,[10,11] or local nerve root/cord compression with consequent paralysis,[12] are reviewed in detail, and a pamphlet we have prepared with literature about the procedure is given to every patient to take home.

■ Imaging Evaluation

Plain films, computed tomography (CT) scan, bone scan, and magnetic resonance imaging (MRI) are all considered complementary to some degree in the evaluation of compression fractures; however, we consider MRI the modality of choice. Advantages inherent in MRI include the greater soft tissue resolution as well as, with the implementation of

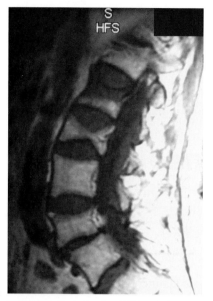
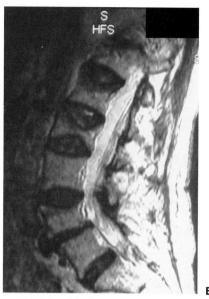
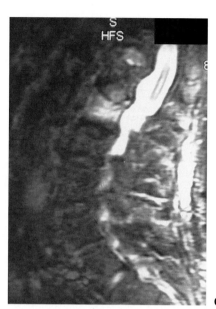

FIGURE 5–1 Sagittal T1-weighted image **(A)** demonstrates multiple lumbar compression fractures with hypointensity involving superior aspect of L1. T2-weighted image **(B)** demonstrates no significant corresponding increased marrow signal but this becomes obvious on STIR sequence **(C)**, indicating acuity.

short-time inversion recovery (STIR), or other fat-suppressing sequences, the ability to differentiate acute from more chronic and stable fractures. These fat-suppressing sequences allow differentiation between marrow edema and the otherwise normal high signal of fatty marrow on standard turbo spin echo (TSE) T2-weighted sequences. On MRI, an acute fracture exhibits T1 hypointensity representing edema of normally high marrow signal (Fig. **5–1**). If there is suspicion of pathologic fracture (malignancy) such as signal abnormality involving the pedicle, or unexpected soft tissue component, a core biopsy can be taken contemporaneously.

It should be kept in mind that although bone scans are useful in those patients for whom MRI is contraindicated (most commonly because of an implanted cardiac pacemaker), there can be abnormal increased uptake as long as osteoclastic activity continues, which can be up to 2 years following a fracture. In those patients with multiple compression fractures of varying age, the clinical exam and sequential plain films demonstrating acuteness become critical for proper evaluation (Fig. **5–2**). Correlative CT scanning with reformatting is critical for evaluation of the paraspinal anatomy and the exclusionary criteria given above.

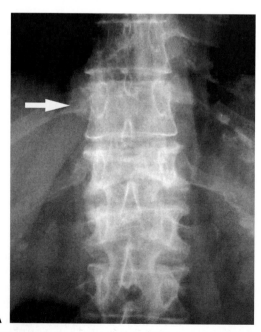
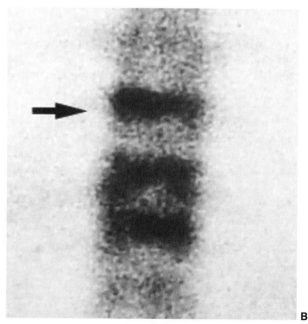

FIGURE 5–2 Anteroposterior (AP) thoracolumbar junction plain film **(A)** reveals compression fractures of T12, L1, and L2, all of which are chronic. Bone scan **(B)**, however, demonstrated unexpected uptake at T11 (arrows), explaining the patient's acute pain.

■ Materials

Needles

An 11-gauge 10-cm bone biopsy needle (Cook Incorporated, Bloomington, IN) (Fig. **5–3A**) is usually selected. In cases where small pedicles preclude use of an 11-gauge needle, we choose the thinner, 13-gauge needle. Extra length may be necessary for large body habitus as well as for a far lateral (rather than the usual transpedicular) approach, in which case a 15-cm needle is selected. If a concomitant core bone biopsy is contemplated, our needle of choice is a 17-gauge, 15-cm Percucut needle (E-Z-EM, Inc., Westbury, NY). This needle has a self-threading

mechanism to gain the core and can be used coaxially with either larger Cook needle (Fig. **5–3B-D**).

Polymethylmethacrylate Mixture

We use the Codman Cranioplast kit (CMW Laboratories, Blackpool, England) (Fig. **5–3E,F**). This material is used in many operations such as cranioplasty and innumerable orthopedic procedures. The material consists of a powdered polymer, which is activated by the addition of a liquid monomer. In our practice, of the 30 g of powder that are supplied, about 1 teaspoon of powder is excluded and the remainder is mixed with 6 g barium sulfate for opacification, and 1.2 g of tobramycin

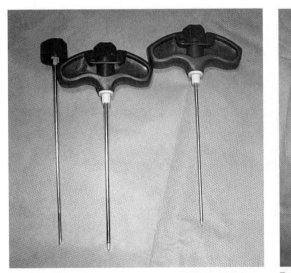
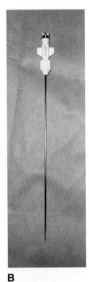
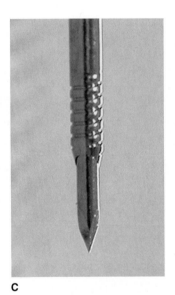
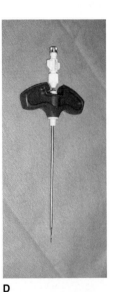

A   **B**   **C**   **D**

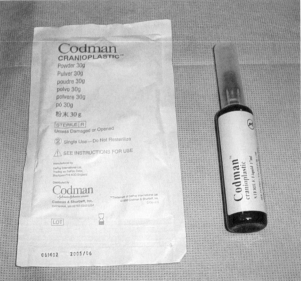
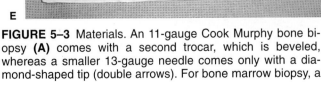

E

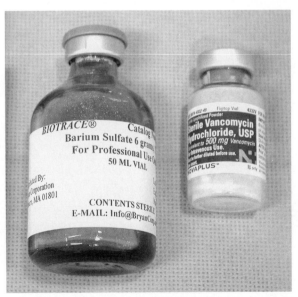

F

FIGURE 5–3 Materials. An 11-gauge Cook Murphy bone biopsy **(A)** comes with a second trocar, which is beveled, whereas a smaller 13-gauge needle comes only with a diamond-shaped tip (double arrows). For bone marrow biopsy, a 17-gauge Percucut needle **(B)** with a self-threading mechanism **(C)** is utilized in a coaxial fashion **(D)**. Codman cranioplast powder **(E)** (left) is mixed with liquid monomer **(E)** (right), barium powder **(F)**

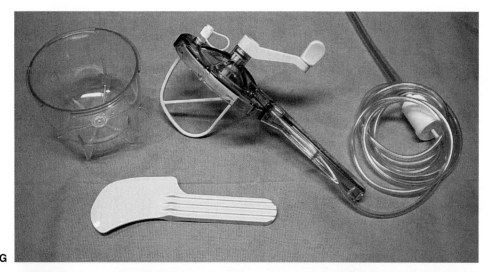

G

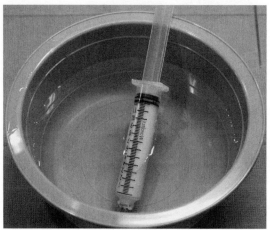

H   I

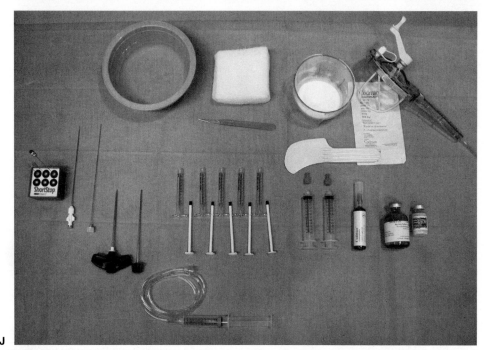

J

FIGURE 5–3 (*Continued*) (left) and vancomycin powder **(F)** (right) in an Ultramix mixing chamber **(G)**. When a glaze-like consistency **(H)** is achieved, it is drawn up into 10-cc syringes, capped, and placed in an ice bath **(I)**. Our standard table setup is shown **(J)**.

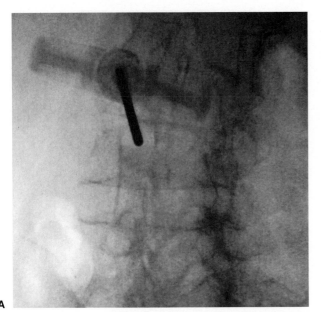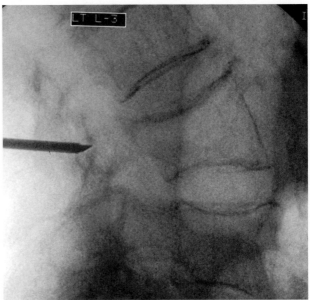

A   B

FIGURE 5–4 AP **(A)** and lateral **(B)** planes are adjusted to maximize visualization of the pedicle and neural foramen, respectively.

(Nebcin, Eli Lilly, Indianapolis, IN) or (because of recent availability issues) 500 mg of vancomycin powder for infection control (Fig. **5–3F**). The liquid monomer is added, and well mixed in an Ultramix mixing chamber (Depuy International Ltd., Blackpool, England) (Fig. **5–3G**).

When a thin "cake-glaze" consistency (Fig. **5–3H**) is achieved, the material is drawn up into 10-mL syringes, capped and immediately kept in an iced saline bath (Fig. **5–3I**). We earlier reported that PMMA polymerization time can be extended so that it is injectable even beyond 2 hours by simply placing it in an ice bath.[13] Our standard table setup is shown in Fig. **5–3J**).

■ Basic Vertebroplasty Technique

Vertebroplasty is performed in an angiography suite under sterile conditions. After completing the informed consent process, the patient is placed in the prone position on the angiography table. Some authors have reported the usefulness of CT guidance, especially in the extremely osteoporotic patient in whom landmarks are difficult to ascertain or in those with small pedicles. However, we have not experienced such limitations and have been able to treat all cases with biplane fluoroscopy.

All patients have continuous physiologic monitoring under monitored anesthesia care. This allows us to concentrate on the actual procedure while the anesthetist takes care of sedation issues. Initially, the angle of anteroposterior fluoroscopy is adjusted as to maximize the oval-like appearance of the target pedicle (Fig. **5–4A**).

Next, on lateral fluoroscopy positioning (Fig. **5–4B**), there should be maximal visualization of the pedicle, neural foramen, and posterior aspect of the vertebral body. It often helps to align the vertebral bodies adjacent to the fractured one to obtain maximum information.

Following the usual sterile preparation, the skin, soft tissues, and periosteum of the targeted pedicle are anesthetized with 1% lidocaine, after sterile preparation of the puncture site. Initially, a 20-gauge spinal needle is positioned, as a guide, with its tip in the center of the pedicle (Fig. **5–5A**). A small skin incision (5 mm) is then made using a No. 11 scalpel. Next, maintaining the same trajectory as the spinal needle, the 11-gauge bone biopsy needle is advanced, such that its tip overlies the center of the oval on anteroposterior (AP) fluoroscopy and in the appropriate position in the lateral plane (Fig. **5–5B,C**). Here, the needle tip should ideally be positioned along the line drawn through the middle of the pedicle. The needle is advanced carefully, under biplane fluoroscopy, and any fine adjustments can be made. A beveled tip, which is available with the 11-gauge needle, can be helpful in "bevel-guiding" the needle to its intended target position within the vertebral body (Fig. **5–5D**). In the case of osteoporotic compression fractures, if the needle is placed correctly, one should encounter only mild resistance to advancement with finger pressure only, which is often required for advancement. The compressed portions of the vertebral body, however, may require significant effort to advance especially in cases of osteoblastic lesions. On rare occasion we have resorted to using an orthopedic hammer.

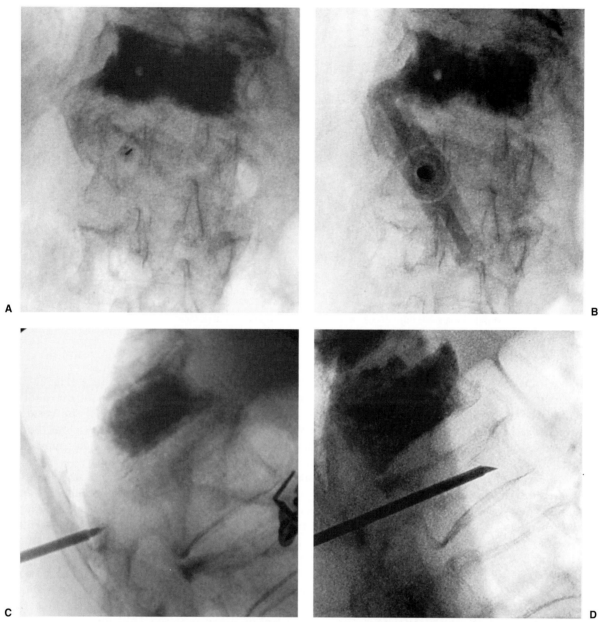

FIGURE 5–5 A 20-gauge spinal needle or smaller anesthetiz-ing needle is used as a target guide **(A)** for subsequent 11-gauge needle placement **(B,C)** into the junction of the pedicle and vertebral body. In the bevel guiding technique, to encourage needle placement inferiorly, the stylet is changed to a beveled edge to "steer" it to the intended target at the junc-tion of the anterior and middle thirds of the vertebral body **(D)**.

Using the lateral plane, the tip of the needle is ad-vanced to the junction of the anterior and middle thirds of the vertebral body (Fig. **5–5D**). The stylet is removed and an epidural venogram obtained prior to injecting cement. This requires a minimum of additional time, contrast, and radiation; only 2 to 3 cc of contrast are required to ac-quire the necessary information. It has been argued that cement and contrast, because of their different viscosities, may not follow the same path; we have found venography to be critical in identifying rapid venous egress either to the epidural venous plexus, directly into inferior

vena cava (IVC) or to paraspinal veins (Fig. **5–6A,B**). This enables us to anticipate leakage point origins from where there may be potential for early pulmonary em-bolization (Fig. **5–6C**) or epidural leakage. If high flow is identified, the needle tip may be advanced slightly. In all our patients venography is performed, to minimize these aforementioned risks of the procedure.

After venography, the PMMA cement is mixed. Our PMMA, as described above, is formed in an Ultramix chamber, which is attached to a vacuum to minimize aerosolization of the liquid monomer. It is mixed until a

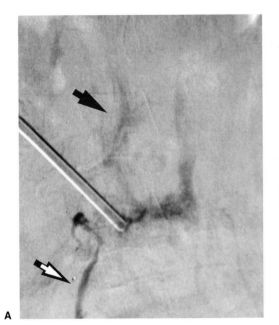

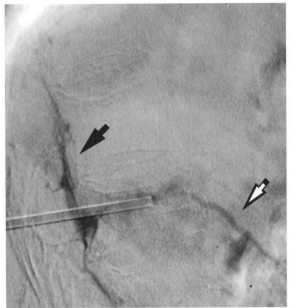

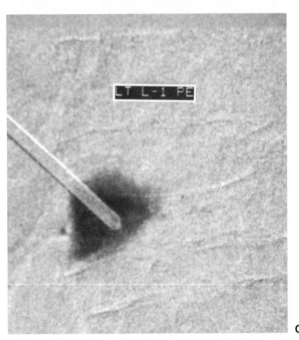

FIGURE 5–6 Venogram. The typical intraosseous pattern is identified in the AP **(A)** and lateral **(B)** planes. In addition, there is visualization of a paraspinal vein (open arrow) and epidural veins (solid arrows), which may predict the subsequent possible path of cement. Being aware of this potential danger allows one to minimize errant cement placement. The road-mapped image demonstrates a trace amount of cement seen in the same paraspinal vein **(C)** (arrowhead); therefore, cement deposition is stopped until the polymethylmethacrylate (PMMA) hardens in the vein, following which more cement may be injected without risk of pulmonary emboli.

shiny cake-glaze consistency is obtained and then drawn up into 10-cc syringes, capped, and kept in an iced saline bath.

One-milliliter reinforced-stem Luer-lock syringes (Fig. **5–7**) are then back-loaded with PMMA from the 10-mL syringes, and are attached tightly to the hub of the bone biopsy needle in place. Injection is then begun under biplane fluoroscopy with road-mapping for increased sensitivity of cement visualization (Fig. **5–8A,B**). About 0.1- to 0.3-mL aliquots of the PMMA mix is repeatedly injected with immediate road-map checks. Careful observation is required of its movement through the bone, and the injection must be stopped when any extraosseous filling is noted. It is especially necessary to pay close attention when the cement is noted to come into the posterior third of the vertebral body for it is after this that increased risk of basivertebral plexus egress into the epidural venous system becomes a real potential. Migration of PMMA into the epidural veins can cause compression of the nerve root or the spinal cord. The caliber of the central canal at the level of injection is critical a priori information gained from previous cross-sectional imaging. Injection is continued until contralateral filling is achieved, or extravasation into veins or paravertebral region is seen. The needle is removed, and the contralateral side is treated in the same way if

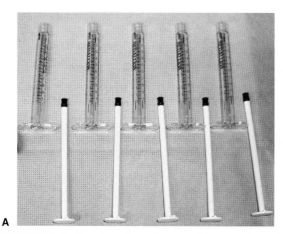
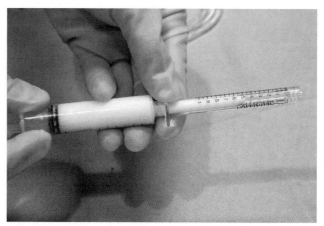

FIGURE 5–7 The 1-cc, Luer-lock reinforced-stem syringes **(A)** are back-loaded with cement **(B)**.

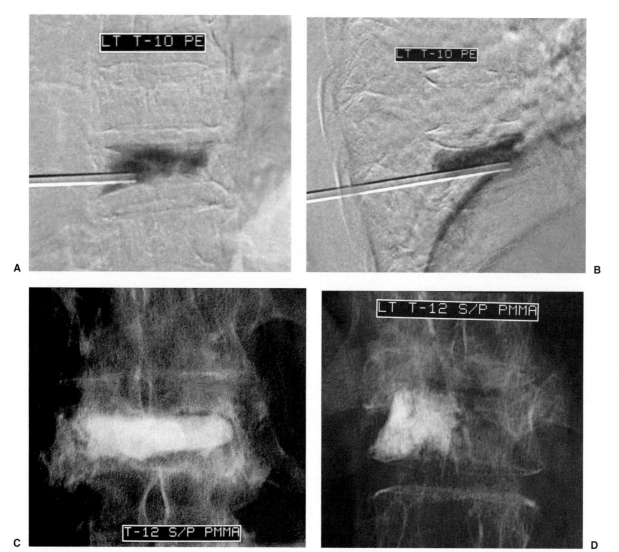

FIGURE 5–8 Using fluoroscopic road-mapping, cement is injected and observed in both the AP **(A)** and lateral **(B)** planes to fill the vertebral body. In this instance the entire vertebral body is filled from a unilateral approach **(C)**.

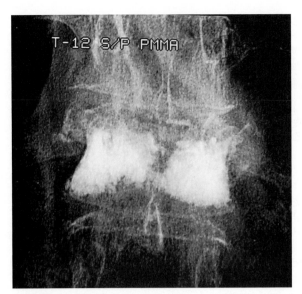

FIGURE 5–8 (*Continued*) Usually, a bilateral approach is necessary **(D,E)**.

inadequate filling occurred from the initial cement deposition (Fig. **5–8C–E**). Once the injection is stopped, the needle is immediately removed both to minimize chances of infection and to avoid hardening of a core within the needle with subsequent filling of the needle track to the skin. As the needle is removed, one should check that this does not occur. Again, road-mapped imaging helps in noting if a core of cement is being left along the tract, and if it is, it can be broken at the posterior margin of the pedicle at the soft tissue interface.

More than two levels of vertebroplasty are treatable at the same sitting, depending on the patient's condition and tolerance. We have injected up to five levels in one stage. After final needle removal, the puncture sites are cleaned and dressed with sterile dressing and Betadine ointment.

Following the procedure, all patients are placed in the supine position for 2 hours, and after this period are allowed to sit or stand as tolerated. Most patients are able to return to their home the same day of the procedure; if very elderly with significant comorbidities, we usually admit overnight on a medical floor. Patients are encouraged to minimize use of pain medications following the procedure. If on long-term narcotics, a taper is immediately begun.

■ Posterolateral Approach

Some patients have very small pedicles precluding use of an 11-gauge needle. In these patients, it is not possible to use a routine transpedicular approach. CT guidance may be useful to treat such patients; however, this method is somewhat cumbersome, requiring both fluoroscopy and CT scan in the procedure room, complicating the procedure. In this case, we use a thinner, 13-gauge needle and utilize a posterolateral approach. In this method we use a more lateral starting point, and traverse the lateral process, thereby reaching the vertebral body more anteriorly (Fig. **5–9**). This method is not especially difficult, and it is less risky because fewer dangerous structures exist along this course.

Both routine transpedicular and posterolateral approaches are diagrammatically summarized in Fig. **5–10**.

■ Biopsy

If there is a suspicion of malignancy or other pathology, a biopsy can be performed at the same time as the vertebroplasty. We place a 10-cm, 11-gauge Cook needle near the junction of the pedicle and vertebral body and utilize a 17-gauge Percucut needle system to obtain core

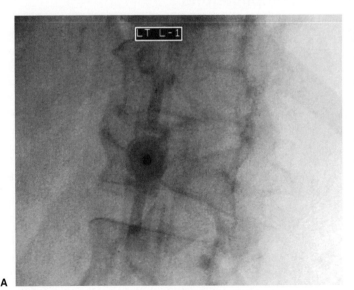
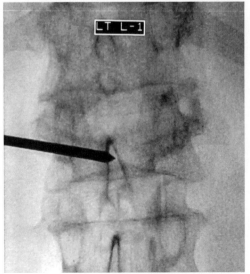

FIGURE 5–9 Using a posterolateral approach (see text), a more anteromedial needle placement can be achieved **(A,B)**.

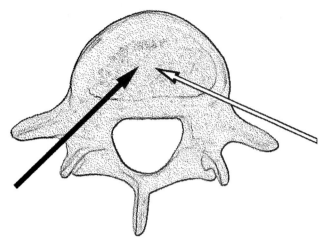

FIGURE 5-10 Diagrammatic summary of transpedicular (solid arrow) and posterolateral (open arrow) approaches.

biopsies from the pedicle and vertebral body proper (Fig. **5-11**).

■ Results

From September 1998 to September 2002, a total of 255 patients underwent percutaneous vertebroplasty in our department; 489 levels of vertebral bodies in 327 procedures were performed on these patients. The mean age of the patients was 75.3 years, with a range of 39 to 99 years. There were 49 men and 206 women; 199 patients

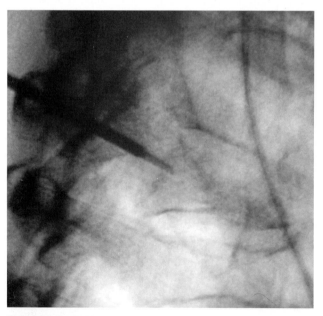

FIGURE 5-11 When the needle is at the pedicle–body junction, the biopsy can be performed using a coaxial system. Here a 17-gauge Percucut core biopsy needle is utilized during percutaneous vertebroplasty.

TABLE 5-1 Summary of Vertebroplasty Results in 224 Follow-Up Patients

	Male	Female	Total
Complete pain relief	20 (47.6%)	93 (51.1%)	113 (50.4%)
Partial pain relief	18 (42.9%)	66 (36.3%)	84 (37.5%)
No pain relief	4 (9.5%)	23 (12.6%)	27 (12.1%)
Worsening of pain	0 (0%)	0 (0%)	0 (0%)
Total	42	182	224

(78%) were treated in one procedure, 46 patients (18%) underwent percutaneous vertebroplasty twice, seven patients (2.7%) were treated three times, one patient (0.4%) was treated four times, one patient (0.4%) was treated five times, and one patient (0.4%) was treated six times. The number of compression fractures were as follows: One vertebral body was treated in 121 patients, two vertebral bodies were treated in 81 patients, three in 25 patients, four in 17 patients, five in six patients, six in three patients, seven in one patient, and eight in one patient. Of these, we treated 221 thoracic compression fractures and 268 lumbar. The number of levels treated in one session were one in 191 patients, two in 117 patients, three in 16 patients, four in two patients, and five in one patient. The amount of PMMA injected per vertebral body varied from 1.0 to 22.0 mL, with an average injection amount of 7.81 mL. Regarding pain relief, 197 (87.9%) of 224 follow-up patients described it as complete (50.4%) or partial (37.5%). Of these, 42 were male and 182 were female. Nonresponders numbered 27 (12.1%); four were male and 23 were female. No patient encountered worsening of pain. This is summarized in Table **5-1**.

■ Complications

The complication rate of the procedure has been reported in some series, ranging from 0 to 10%. The primary reported neurologic complication is leakage of PMMA through the fracture lines, the needle tract, or the epidural venous complex, causing spinal cord or nerve root compression.[12] Nonneurologic complications have been described including symptomatic (and lethal) pulmonary embolism,[10,11] transient systemic hypotension apparently from monomer toxicity,[14] infection, and rib fractures.[8] Leakage of cement into the disk space is a relatively common occurrence, indicating the fracture site has been reached; unless there is significant disk bulge or protrusion, this is usually asymptomatic. We have not experienced problems related to this; however, if potential disk resection is contemplated, cement may make the surgery technically more difficult. This scenario should be considered in patient management.

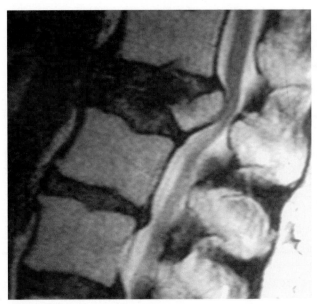 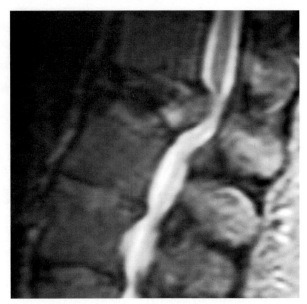

A   B

FIGURE 5–12 Example of a retropulsed bone fragment in an acute fracture considered a contraindication for vertebroplasty. **(A)** T2-weighted image. **(B)** STIR.

In our series, we had one patient with a burst fracture (similar to the patient in Fig. **5–12**) develop foot drop in a delayed fashion about 2 weeks after the procedure, but there were no other neurologic complications. This complication occurred early in our experience, and we subsequently made this an exclusion criterion for vertebroplasty in our practice. We have had no instances of symptomatic pulmonary embolism, infection, or monomer toxicity. Because of our ability to detect small quantities of epidural and paraspinal leak early, we have had no symptomatic complications.

■ Conclusion

In our experience percutaneous vertebroplasty is an extremely effective and safe method for achieving pain relief and conferring an element of structural stability to the patient's spine. Very few procedures in medicine have this degree of success and level of patient satisfaction. With excellent quality imaging, complications appear to be rare. Percutaneous vertebroplasty shows great promise, with improving techniques and the development of more biocompatible cements.

REFERENCES

1. Galibert P, Deramond H, Rosat P, Le Gars D. Note preliminaire sur le traitement des angiomes vertebraux par vertebroplastie acrylique percutanee. Neurochirurgie 1987;33:166–168
2. Amar AP, Larsen DW, Esnaashari N, Albuquerque FC, Lavine SD, Teitelbaum GP. Percutaneous transpedicular polymethylmethacrylate vertebroplasty for the treatment of spinal compression fractures. Neurosurgery 2001;49:1105–1114
3. Barr JD, Barr MS, Lemley TJ, McCann RM. Percutaneous vertebroplasty for pain relief and spinal stabilization. Spine 2000;25:923–928
4. Cortet B, Cotten A, Boutry N, et al. Percutaneous vertebroplasty in the treatment of osteoporotic vertebral compression fractures: an open prospective study. J Rheumatol 1999;26:2222–2228
5. Cyteval C, Sarrabere MP, Roux JO, et al. Acute osteoporotic vertebral collapse: open study on percutaneous injection of acrylic surgical cement in 20 patients. AJR Am J Roentgenol 1999;173:1685–1690
6. Deramond H, Depriester C, Galibert P, Le Gars D. Percutaneous vertebroplasty with polymethylmethacrylate: technique, indications, and results. Radiol Clin North Am 1998;36:533–546
7. Grados F, Depriester C, Cayrolle G, Hardy N, Deramond H, Fardellone P. Long-term observations of vertebral osteoporotic fractures treated by percutaneous vertebroplasty. Rheumatology (Oxford) 2000;39:1410–1414
8. Jensen ME, Evans AJ, Mathis JM, Kallmes DF, Cloft HJ, Dion JE. Percutaneous polymethylmethacrylate vertebroplasty in the treatment of osteoporotic vertebral body compression fractures: technical aspects. AJNR Am J Neuroradiol 1997;18:1897–1904
9. Jensen ME, Dion JE. Percutaneous vertebroplasty in the treatment of osteoporotic compression fractures. Neuroimaging Clin North Am 2000;10:547–568
10. Bernhard J, Heini PF, Villiger PM. Asymptomatic diffuse pulmonary embolism cause by acrylic cement: an unusual complication of percutaneous vertebroplasty. Ann Rheum Dis 2003;62:85–86
11. Jang JS, Lee SH, Jung SK. Pulmonary embolism of polymethylmethacrylate after percutaneous vertebroplasty: a report of three cases. Spine 2002;27:E416–418
12. Lee BJ, Lee SR, Yoo TY. Paraplegia as a complication of percutaneous vertebroplasty with polymethylmethacrylate: a case report. Spine 2002;27:E419–422
13. Chavali RV, Resijeck R, Knight SK, Choi IS. Extending Polymerization time of polymethylmethacrylate cement in percutaneous vertebroplasty with ice bath cooling. AJNR Am J Neuroradiol 2003;24:545–546
14. Vasconcelos C, Gailloud P, Beauchamp NJ, Heck DV, Murphy KJ. Is percutaneous vertebroplasty without pretreatment venography safe? Evaluation of 205 consecutives procedures. AJNR Am J Neuroradiol 2002;23:913–917

6

Complication Avoidance and Management in Percutaneous Vertebroplasty

FRANK C. TONG AND JACQUES E. DION

Objectives: On completion of this chapter, the reader should be able to describe the historical differences between vertebroplasty and kyphoplasty.

Accreditation: The American Association of Neurological Surgeons is accredited by the Accreditation Council for Continuing Medical Education to sponsor continuing medical education for physicians.

Credit: The American Association of Neurological Surgeons designates this continuing medical education activity for a maximum of 15 credits in Category I of the Physician's Recognition Award of the American Medical Association.

The Home Study Examination is online at www.aans.org/education/books/vertebro.asp

Since percutaneous vertebroplasty was first described in 1987[1] there has been progressive evolution in the technique, materials, and even types of patients who are now treated using this technique. Along with its well-documented clinical effectiveness and minimally invasive approach, one of the strengths of this treatment has been a very low complication rate. Complications from percutaneous vertebroplasty fall into a continuum where small amounts of cement placed in the epidural soft tissues, adjacent intervertebral disks, or epidural veins will likely remain clinically silent, whereas larger amounts of material in these identical locations can cause symptoms of radicular pain, spinal cord compression, pulmonary embolus, or even stroke.

The overall incidence of clinically significant complication following percutaneous vertebroplasty is low, ranging from 1 to 10% in various series. These include worsening pain, iatrogenic fracture, infection, neurologic compromise, and pulmonary embolus. With proper attention to patient selection and technique, the risk of subsequent symptomatic complication can be minimized. Table **6–1** summarizes the incidence of these symptomatic complications for both osteoporotic and pathologic fractures for some larger, recently published series.

The great majority (>90%) of fractures treated in these series were of osteoporotic origin. When examined separately, percutaneous vertebroplasty for malignant fractures demonstrates a significantly higher incidence of symptomatic complications, ranging from 5 to 10%. Pathologic fractures are typically more difficult to treat and commonly demonstrate irregular polymethyl-methacrylate (PMMA) filling patterns and higher incidence of cement leakage into the epidural veins. This may be at least partially attributable to the higher incidence of posterior vertebral body cortical compromise in patients with malignant fractures. However, most of the pathologic fracture treatment data are also older, reflecting a period when there was overall less experience with this technique. This subset of patients is summarized in Table **6–2**.

This chapter addresses the prevention and management of symptomatic complications at each stage of the procedure. Accurate needle placement and the quantity of cement lost during injection primarily affect whether a patient may manifest imaging findings of a small cement leakage or subsequently develop undesirable clinical symptoms. It is therefore of the utmost importance to comprehensively visualize and understand the anatomy and to pay meticulous attention to technique. This enables the operator to rapidly recognize and address undesirable needle or cement placement in the earliest stages, thereby decreasing the likelihood of clinical complications.

TABLE 6–1 Overall Incidence of Clinical Complications Following Percutaneous Vertebroplasty

	Jensen 1997[2]	Barr 2000[3]	Amar 2001[4]	Kallmes 2002[5]	McGraw 2002[6]	Vasconcelos 2002[7]
Number of patients	29	47	97	41	100	137
Number of levels	47	84	258	63	156	205
Infection	0	0	0	1	0	0
Radicular compromise	0	1	2 radicular pain symptoms, 1 quadriceps weakness from root compression	0	1 radicular symptom	1 radicular symptom from cement through lateral wall dehiscence
Epidural compromise	0	0	1 clonus (3 asymptomatic)	0	0	0
Pulmonary embolism	0	0	3 (2 asymptomatic, 1 symptomatic)	0	0	1? (not symptomatic)
Rib/pedicle fracture	2 rib	0	0	1 pedicle	0	0
Other		1 nonbacterial urethritis from catheter placement	2 deaths from pneumonia and delayed brainstem stroke, 1 dural tear, 1 fever and atelectasis from general anesthesia, 1 transient hypotension		1 sternal fracture during patient transfer	1 transient hypotension, 1 puncture site dysesthesia

■ Patient Selection

Persistent or Worsening Pain

The selection process is a primary determinant of whether a patient will experience significant pain relief following the procedure. Careful review and localization of the patient's symptoms, imaging, and medical history are crucial to minimizing persistent or worsening symptoms of pain. Potential screening and localization pitfalls include misidentification of the symptomatic level

TABLE 6–2 Incidence of Clinical Symptoms Following Percutaneous Vertebroplasty in Patients with Spinal Malignancy

	Chiras 1995[8]	Weill 1996[9]	Cotten 1996[10]	Jang 2002[11]
Number of patients	113	37	37	27
Number of levels	120	52	40	72
Infection	1	0	0	0
Radicular compromise	10	3	2	0
Epidural compromise	1	0	0	0
Pulmonary embolism		0	0	2
Rib/pedicle fracture		0	0	
Other		2 transient difficulty swallowing	1 transient femoral neuropathy following leak into psoas muscle	

or extracorporeal sources of pain that will not improve following cementation of the vertebral body. These potential extracorporeal sources include pain arising from spinal stenosis, degenerative facet disease, posterior element fracture, and disk disease.

It is therefore important to corroborate both the clinical and the imaging findings to specifically identify those levels responsible for the patient's symptoms. This may include additional imaging modalities such as palpation of individual vertebral bodies under fluoroscopy, bone scan with single photon emission computed tomography (SPECT), computed tomography (CT), or magnetic resonance imaging (MRI). The presence of marrow edema on MRI is suggestive of fracture acuity, whereas bone scan and SPECT imaging can be very helpful in identifying "active" vertebral body lesions or fractures involving the posterior elements. Commonly, the patient may experience pain from multiple fractures, which can be treated either at one sitting or sequentially in a staged treatment approach.

■ Needle Placement

Bleeding or Dural Tear

Cement delivery in vertebroplasty requires percutaneous placement of an 11- of 13-gauge needle into the compressed vertebral body. Potential associated complications during needle placement include bleeding, hematoma, neurologic injury, pedicle fracture, and infection. The risk of bleeding complication can be minimized by ensuring that the patient's coagulation factors [prothrombin time (PT), partial thromboplastin time (PTT), international normalized ratio (INR), and platelets] are normal in addition to carefully maintaining a transpedicular needle placement approach. Violation of the medial margin of the pedicle by the needle can cause tearing of the thecal sac[12] and injury to the spinal cord or nerve roots, in addition to epidural, subdural, or subarachnoid hemorrhage. Therefore, adequate visualization of the pedicle is absolutely crucial during needle placement.

Pedicle or Rib Fracture

Care should also be taken not to torque the needle excessively during placement to minimize the chances of iatrogenic pedicle fracture. Alignment of the needle bevel can be helpful in changing the direction of the needle tip without transmitting excessive force to the pedicle. Rib fractures in osteoporotic patients have also been noted secondary to forces transmitted to the rib cage with the patient prone during needle placement. The use of a small orthopedic hammer during needle placement may ultimately diminish the risk of iatrogenic rib fracture. Both rib fractures and pedicle fractures are typically managed conservatively.

Infection

Adherence to sterile operative technique is required to minimize the chances of subsequent infection. Common adjunctive means of further decreasing the risk of infection include administration of systemic antibiotics and adding tobramycin to the vertebroplasty cement. Tobramycin remains effective following the exothermic cement curing and subsequently leaches out of the cement over time, providing local coverage. Review of the literature demonstrates only two documented cases of infection following percutaneous vertebroplasty, although there have been anecdotal reports of others. It should be noted that infection can occur despite administration of both prophylactic systemic antibiotics and tobramycin in the PMMA. In the two published cases, infection eventually cleared with intravenous antibiotic therapy.[5,8] Vertebral osteomyelitis is a very serious complication that may require corpectomy and carries up to a 50% mortality risk in the geriatric population.

■ Venogram

Contrast Allergy

Venography is often performed to assess the location of the needle tip relative to the draining veins prior to cement injection. If the venogram demonstrates prominent early venous filling, the operator may elect to reposition the needle tip or mix the cement with greater viscosity to minimize epidural venous filling and therefore decrease the risk of pulmonary embolus. The risks associated with venography include a very small percentage of contrast allergy with symptoms including urticaria, rash, hives, laryngospasm, or profound hypotension. Fortunately, the incidence of life-threatening contrast reaction is rare, and a patient with a history of urticaria, rash, or hives following contrast administration should be pretreated with oral steroids. Patients with severe contrast reactions such as laryngospasm or profound systemic hypotension should not undergo contrast venography.

There has been debate regarding whether venography is necessary or useful in percutaneous vertebroplasty. The potential benefit for inexperienced operators is that it functions as a road map to the venous anatomy, demonstrating sites of potential venous cement leakage. Early and prompt filling of the epidural veins has also prompted some operators to prophylactically embolize these veins with Avitene or Gelfoam slurry.

■ Cement Preparation

Infection

The structural integrity of vertebroplasty cement is largely dependent on proper mixing and ratios of the various components. These include the powdered and liquid components of the PMMA, opacifying barium, and tobramycin. The inclusion of tobramycin in the cement mixture provides local levels of antibiotic following the procedure, which likely helps to decrease the risk of procedural infection. Overall, the inclusion of tobramycin in the PMMA solution does not appear to significantly affect cement strength. To date, there have been no published hypersensitivity reactions to tobramycin in the PMMA preparation.

Cement Fracture and Hypersensitivity

The relative viscosity of the PMMA mixture can be adjusted by increasing or decreasing the relative amount of liquid monomer in solution. Mixing the PMMA to a more liquid state can enhance the penetration of the cement throughout the vertebral body, with the potential disadvantage of earlier filling of epidural veins increasing the risk or neurologic compromise and symptomatic pulmonary embolism. Laboratory studies have also demonstrated up to 24% weakening of the cured cement when monomer is added at higher or lower ratios than recommended by the cement manufacturer.[13] In addition, there have been a few cases of apparent hypersensitivity to the

PMMA in which patients develop acute postprocedural fevers lasting 24 to 36 hours that resolve spontaneously. These are managed successfully with antipyretics such as acetaminophen or ibuprofen. The self-limiting and hyperacute nature of these fevers in the absence of white blood count (WBC) elevation suggest that these represent hypersensitivity reactions rather than infection.

Epidural Vein Filling and Incomplete Opacification

Barium is a necessary opacifying agent for the otherwise nonradiopaque PMMA. Inadequate amounts of barium (<30%) within the mixture make it difficult for the operator to visualize the material during injection, which increases the risk of undesirable cement deposition in the epidural veins or the lungs. Although increasing the relative concentration of barium beyond recommended levels may help to further enhance the visibility of the PMMA, bench studies show that there is significant decrease in the cement strength once this increases beyond a 30% concentration. The author knows of one patient who suffered a subsequent cement fracture through a previously vertebroplastied level where the operator used approximately twice the recommended amount of barium, thus compromising the structural integrity of the material.

■ Cement Injection

The injection of PMMA into the vertebral body under imaging guidance is the step that offers the most opportunity for clinically significant complication. These include passage of PMMA through the epidural veins to the lungs, causing symptomatic pulmonary embolus and cement in the basivertebral plexus and epidural veins, causing compression of the spinal cord or nerve roots, or thermal injury to the anterior spinal artery or spinal cord. Pressure should not be allowed to accumulate unchecked within the injection syringe or injection device, as the PMMA can abruptly migrate into the epidural veins. Adjustment of the needle position may be required to place the cement in the marrow space and away from the draining veins.

Transient Hypotension

Although transient hypotension is more commonly reported with PMMA injection in hip arthroplasty, clinical hypotension has been rarely described with percutaneous vertebroplasty.[14] Possible causes include fat emboli from the marrow, hypersensitivity to cement monomer, and reflex autonomic response from increased intramedullary pressure during PMMA injection.[15]

Clinical hypotension is a rare finding, with some authors disputing the association between PMMA injection and systemic cardiovascular derangement.[16]

Acrylic Cement Embolus

There have been no published reports of patient deaths following percutaneous vertebroplasty. However, there have been anecdotal reports of two patients who died following multilevel vertebroplasties with large-volume cement injections. These patients were found to have large amounts of PMMA deposited in the pulmonary arteries, resulting in fatal pulmonary embolus, and these procedures were performed under general anesthesia where the operator apparently did not recognize the loss of cement to the epidural veins and lungs.

Adequate opacification of the PMMA and visualization of the material and the spinal anatomy during injection are absolutely critical. Venography may be useful for identification of venous anatomy; venogram images can be stored as reference images on one of the fluoroscope monitors for the detection of small amounts of cement escape during injection. Because it is not possible to aspirate errant cement, close attention must be paid to fluoroscopic technique and projection so that epidural cement can be recognized as early as possible and the injection terminated or paused. If cement is identified in an epidural space before the vertebral body is adequately filled, the injection can be paused for a few minutes, allowing the cement in the veins to partially cure. Resumption of injection frequently causes new cement to further fill the vertebral body as access to these partially filled epidural veins becomes blocked by cured material.

Pulmonary Embolus

Pulmonary embolus resulting from cement extrusion is an uncommon event that can be difficult to detect clinically during cement injection. In one series 3 of 97 patients developed pulmonary embolism with only one experiencing subsequent pulmonary edema and shortness of breath following the procedure.[4] The remaining two patients were asymptomatic. None of the three patients developed notable changes in their oxygen saturation during cement injection. There is one published case of symptomatic pulmonary acrylic cement embolism causing hypoxia and pulmonary infarction presenting clinically hours after the procedure with pain and hypoxia that was managed with anticoagulants and supplemental oxygen with ultimate resolution of symptoms.[17] Additionally, three of 27 patients treated for spinal malignancy developed pulmonary emboli, with two of them manifesting clinical symptoms that were also successfully treated with anticoagulation and supplemental oxygen.[11] The authors of this series attributed the incidence of pulmonary embolus to an overly thin PMMA mixture, resulting in higher losses of material to the paravertebral veins.

Stroke

The presence of a right-to-left circulatory shunt, such as a patent foramen ovale, predisposes a patient to potential complication from stroke as published following a case of intraoperative vertebroplasty.[18]

Neurologic Compromise

The overall risk of neurologic compromise following percutaneous vertebroplasty is relatively higher for patients treated for malignant fractures compared with those treated for osteoporotic fractures. This is most likely due to the fact that osteoporotic compression fractures are generally able to accept more cement in a medullary cavity that is not filled with tumor cells as in a malignant fracture. Additionally, the integrity of the posterior wall of the vertebral body is more commonly compromised in tumor patients with posterior wall cortical destruction or epidural tumor involvement, resulting in epidural cement leakage in up to 37%.[10] Fortunately, the great majority of these remain asymptomatic as long as the leakage is recognized early and the PMMA injection is halted before significant canal compromise occurs.

The overall strategy for prevention of neurologic compromise again focuses on conscientious visualization of the spine in a true lateral projection with adequate visualization of the cement. Cement filling of the epidural veins or basivertebral plexus can be minimized if it is recognized early and the injection is immediately paused long enough for the delivered cement to partially polymerize. Injection of additional cement can then be carefully resumed with preferential filling away from these structures. Termination of injection before the cement approaches the posterior fifth of the vertebral body will also help minimize cement deposition into the anterior epidural space.

Most patients with the infrequent finding of neurologic compromise following percutaneous vertebroplasty present with radicular symptoms rather than symptoms of cord compression. In contrast to epidural cement leakage, foraminal cement deposition is more frequently symptomatic. Radicular symptoms can often be managed with steroids, Neurontin, epidural steroid injection, or nerve block. Patients with intractable symptoms or significant compromise of the spinal canal may ultimately require surgical removal of the polymerized cement.

■ Conclusion

During vertebroplasty, the risk of clinically significant complications such as symptomatic pulmonary embolus, infection, or new neurologic findings following percutaneous vertebroplasty is very low. With careful patient selection and attention to technique, even the inexperienced operator should be able to attain a clinically significant complication risk of <1% for patients with osteoporotic fractures and no more than 5 to 10% for patients with pathologic fractures. Adequate visualization of the spine anatomy, needle tip, and PMMA during the procedure is absolutely crucial to recognizing and preventing potentially serious complications.

For the new practitioner of vertebroplasty, we recommend an initially conservative technique:

1. Bipedicular needle placement
2. Venography to assess epidural drainage pattern
3. Adequate opacification of cement with ~30% barium
4. Relatively low threshold for suspension or termination of cement injection, especially if there is any suspicion of significant cement loss

After becoming more comfortable with the anatomic landmarks and injection technique, it may be possible for the operator to modify this approach without significant change in the operative risk.

REFERENCES

1. Galibert P, Deramond H, Rosat P, Le Gars D. [Preliminary note on the treatment of vertebral angioma by percutaneous acrylic vertebroplasty] (in French). Neurochirurgie 1987;33:166–168
2. Jensen ME, Evans AJ, Mathis JM, Kallmes DF, Cloft HJ, Dion JE. Percutaneous polymethylmethacrylate vertebroplasty in the treatment of osteoporotic vertebral body compression fractures: technical aspects. AJNR Am J Neuroradiol 1997;18:1897–1904
3. Barr JD, Barr MS, Lemley TJ, McCann RM. Percutaneous vertebroplasty for pain relief and spinal stabilization. Spine 2000;25: 923–928
4. Amar AP, Larsen DW, Esnaashari N, Albuquerque FC, Lavine SD, Teitelbaum GP. Percutaneous transpedicular polymethacrylate vertebroplasty for the treatment of spinal compression fractures. Neurosurgery 2001;49:1105–1114; discussion 1114–1115
5. Kallmes DF, Schweickert PA, Marx WF, Jensen ME. Vertebroplasty in the mid- and upper thoracic spine. AJNR Am J Neuroradiol 2002;23:1117–1120
6. McGraw JK, Lippert JA, Minkus KD, Rami PM, Davis TM, Budzik RF. Prospective evaluation of pain relief in 100 patients undergoing percutaneous vertebroplasty: results and follow-up. J Vasc Intervent Radiol 2002;13(9 pt 1):883–886
7. Vasconcelos C, Gailloud P, Beauchamp NJ, Heck DV, Murphy KJ. Is percutaneous vertebroplasty without pretreatment venography safe? Evaluation of 205 consecutives procedures. AJNR Am J Neuroradiol 2002;23:913–917
8. Chiras J, DH. Complications des vertebroplasties. In: Saillant G, ed. Echecs et Complications de la Chirurgie du Rachis. Chirurgie de Reprise. Paris: Sauramps Medical, 1995:149–153

9. Weill A, Chiras J, Simon JM, Rose M, Sola-Martinez T, Enkaoua E. Spinal metastases: indications for and results of percutaneous injection of acrylic surgical cement. Radiology 1996;199:241–247

10. Cotten A, Dewatre F, Cortet B, et al. Percutaneous vertebroplasty for osteolytic metastases and myeloma: effects of the percentage of lesion filling and the leakage of methyl methacrylate at clinical follow-up. Radiology 1996;200:525–530

11. Jang JS, Lee SH, Jung SK. Pulmonary embolism of polymethylmethacrylate after percutaneous vertebroplasty: a report of three cases. Spine 2002;27:E416–E418

12. Gaughen JR Jr, Jensen ME, Schweickert PA, Kaufmann TJ, Marx WF, Kallmes DF. Relevance of antecedent venography in percutaneous vertebroplasty for the treatment of osteoporotic compression fractures. AJNR Am J Neuroradiol 2002;23:594–600

13. Jasper LE, Deramond H, Mathis JM, Belkoff SM. The effect of monomer-to-powder ratio on the material properties of cranioplast. Bone 1999;25(2 suppl):27S–29S

14. Vasconcelos C, Gailloud P, Martin JB, Murphy KJ. Transient arterial hypotension induced by polymethylmethacrylate injection during percutaneous vertebroplasty. J Vasc Intervent Radiol 2001;12:1001–1002

15. Aebli N, Krebs J, Davis G, Walton M, Williams MJ, Theis JC. Fat embolism and acute hypotension during vertebroplasty: an experimental study in sheep. Spine 2002;27:460–466

16. Kaufmann TJ, Jensen ME, Ford G, Gill LL, Marx WF, Kallmes DF. Cardiovascular effects of polymethylmethacrylate use in percutaneous vertebroplasty. AJNR Am J Neuroradiol 2002;23:601–604

17. Padovani B, Kasriel O, Brunner P, Peretti-Viton P. Pulmonary embolism caused by acrylic cement: a rare complication of percutaneous vertebroplasty. AJNR Am J Neuroradiol 1999;20:375–377

18. Scroop R, Eskridge J, Britz GW. Paradoxical cerebral arterial embolization of cement during intraoperative vertebroplasty: case report. AJNR Am J Neuroradiol 2002;23:868–870

7

Patient Selection in the Treatment of Pathologic Compression Fractures

EERIC TRUUMEES AND STEVEN R. GARFIN

Objectives: On completion of this chapter, the reader should be able to describe techniques used for complication avoidance when performing vertebroplasty procedures.

Accreditation: The American Association of Neurological Surgeons is accredited by the Accreditation Council for Continuing Medical Education to sponsor continuing medical education for physicians.

Credit: The American Association of Neurological Surgeons designates this continuing medical education activity for a maximum of 15 credits in Category I of the Physician's Recognition Award of the American Medical Association.

The Home Study Examination is online at www.aans.org/education/books/vertebro.asp

In the United States, there are 700,000 osteoporotic compression fractures per year.[1] Severe back pain attributable to metastatic cancer affects thousands more.[2] Typically, nonoperative treatment controls the pain in the majority of these patients.[3] However, in a large minority, this pain is refractory to conservative measures. The significant morbidity of open operation in these frail patients limits the role of traditional operative techniques.

Even after the pain subsides, many patients are left with a kyphotic deformity. At worst, a chin on chest deformity may develop. In other cases, excessive kyphosis compresses abdominal viscera and lungs, affecting appetite and breathing. Chronic pain from the rib cage on ilium contact or paraspinal muscle spasm is reported.

Recently, augmentation of the vertebral body with polymethylmethacrylate (PMMA) has been described both with fracture reduction (kyphoplasty) and without fracture reduction (vertebroplasty). The early clinical results of vertebral body augmentation (VBA) procedures suggest dramatic decreases in pain and rapid return to function in a large percentage of patients. Yet, to date, no randomized clinical trial of operative versus nonoperative treatment is available for either osteoporotic or neoplastic disease. Moreover, the mechanism of pain relief has not been elucidated.[4]

Patient groups responding well to VBA typically have mechanical incompetence of the target vertebral body. Augmentation of that body with PMMA restores the load-bearing capacity of the vertebral body.[5-7] This restoration of mechanical integrity is thought to relieve pain.[4]

Selecting patients most likely to benefit from kyphoplasty or vertebroplasty is challenging. Accurate identification of the pain generator is critical. The more concordant the history and examination are with the imaging findings, the more likely a successful clinical outcome.

This chapter reviews the indications and contraindications for kyphoplasty and vertebroplasty and discusses the historical, examination, and imaging findings that identify appropriate operative candidates. A clinical approach to the patient with a painful pathologic vertebral body fracture is presented.

■ Operative Indications

In 1987 Galibert and Deramond first described vertebroplasty as a means to treat painful spinal hemangiomas.[8] Later, vertebroplasty of spinal metastases was reported, followed, in 1991, by the first reports of use in benign, osteoporotic compression fractures.[9,10]

TABLE 7–1 Indications for Kyphoplasty and Vertebroplasty: Painful Vertebral Body Fracture from the Following:

Primary osteoporosis
Secondary osteoporosis
Multiple myeloma
Osteolytic metastasis
Osteogenesis imperfecta
Hemangioma

Kyphoplasty, on the other hand, was devised to treat painful osteoporotic compression fractures.[7] Today, aside from certain technical limitations, the indications for both procedures are the same (Table **7–1**). However, there is significant regional variation in the implementation of these techniques.[11] In Europe, for example, metastasis to the spine is a common indication for vertebroplasty, whereas osteoporotic fractures encompass the majority of the North American experience.

Use of kyphoplasty or vertebroplasty for other pathologic entities, such as osteogenesis imperfecta, is undergoing study. Aside from infection, VBA may be considered in any situation wherein mechanical insufficiency of the vertebral body leads to pain and inactivity. However, there are several important limitations and contraindications to the technique.

Osteoporosis

Osteoporosis is a skeletal disorder characterized by compromised bone strength predisposing to an increased risk of fracture (NIH Consensus Conference on Osteoporosis, March 2000). This disorder is typically divided into primary and secondary types. In primary osteoporosis, there is no identifiable cause of the change in bone mass. In secondary osteoporosis, a systemic disorder such as Cushing's disease, hyperthyroidism, or hypogonadism, accelerates bone resorption or impedes bone formation. Decreased bone mass and trabecular interconnectivity decrease the exogenous force required to fracture bones of the axial and appendicular skeleton.

With 700,000 fractures per year, the spine is the most common site of osteoporotic fracture.[1,12,13] The natural history of the fractures, however, is poorly understood. It is difficult to predict the natural history of a given fracture in any patient. Two thirds of these injuries never come to medical attention.[14] Many more resolve with expectant management.[3] Typical, nonoperative management includes pain medications, bracing, and bed rest. However, strict bed rest is associated with a further 4% loss of bone mineral density. This frail patient population is also subject to cardiopulmonary decline and decubitus ulcers while at bed rest.

Thus the first compression fracture leads to functional limitation, which is associated with further bone loss and additional fractures as part of a "vicious cycle."[15] Yet interruption of this cycle by traditional, operative means has been fraught with failure. These patients are often too frail to undergo a major spinal stabilization procedure. When these procedures are attempted, hardware failure in osteoporotic bone increases the risk of poor clinical results. Vertebroplasty and kyphoplasty have been reported to reduce pain and allow earlier return to function, thereby breaking this cycle.

When evaluating osteoporotic patients, it is important to recognize that VBA is only one facet of the appropriate care of the underlying disease process.[16] Several new modalities of bone preservation and restoration including selective estrogen receptor modulators (SERMs) and bisphosphonates have been shown singly, and in combination, to decrease the risk of future fracture.[17–19] Spine surgeons and interventional radiologists typically charged with performing vertebroplasty or kyphoplasty are not well equipped to monitor and treat a patient's underlying osteoporosis.[20] Therefore, a multidisciplinary approach is encouraged.

Treatment of the underlying osteoporosis is especially important given the fear of adjacent segment fracture. Stiff, cemented vertebral bodies may transmit increased compressive loads to neighboring bodies, increasing the risk of new fracture.[21] On the other hand, correction of kyphotic deformity and maintenance of a posterior weight-bearing axis may protect the anterior column. In that the disk space, the least stiff portion of the motion segment, is not affected, changes in load transmission should be minimal. Even in untreated patients, with each fracture, the risk of additional fractures increases.[22]

The osteoporotic patient population may exhibit confounding comorbidities, including advanced spinal degeneration. This spondylosis itself may be a source of pain. Ready identification of painful fractures is complicated by the presence of healed injuries. Finally, nonspinal sources of back pain, such as pancreatic carcinoma and abdominal aortic aneurysm are not unusual in this patient population. Therefore, a complete patient evaluation must be undertaken before recommending VBA.

In well-selected patients, however, excellent outcomes may be expected. Various case series describe significant pain relief in 80 to 97% of patients.[10,23,25,26] This pain relief is typically noted within the first few days after the procedure and has been found to be stable months after the procedure.[24]

Metastasis

Metastasis to the spine is common and often associated with severe pain and disability.[27] Metastases are not themselves directly innervated. Local pain, therefore, is at least partially due to fracture and reaction of the innervated normal bone.[9] In patients with disseminated disease, limited treatment options are available. Surgical extirpation and stabilization is often not indicated due to the wide anatomic range of the disease and the patient's overall frail medical condition.[28]

As in osteoporosis, kyphoplasty and vertebroplasty may decrease pain in subgroups of these patients by providing a sound mechanical environment for load bearing. This mechanical theory for the effectiveness of VBA also explains the inferior results obtained in patients with significant soft tissue extension.[9]

Radiation therapy to a neoplastic compression fracture affords partial or complete relief of symptoms in more than 90%.[29] However, with fractionated dosing, relief may require 2 weeks after the start of therapy. Nonfractionated therapy may accelerate this response.[30,31] After irradiation, the bone does not return to normal mechanical strength. Though a healing response is noted over 2 to 4 months, it has minimal mechanical effect.[30] The recovery of compression strength is thought to be better in myeloma than in solid tumor metastasis.[30] Unfortunately, during this interval, there remains a significant chance of further bony collapse with neurologic compromise (Fig. 7–1).[32] Also, radiation therapy may be

ineffective in those with extensive destruction of the vertebral body.[33]

There are several vertebroplasty series reporting greater than 70% pain relief in patients with metastases to the spine.[9,28,33,34] In one study of 40 patients, 97% had a decrease in pain with a 2 to 3% complication rate and a 1% rate of cord compression. Relief was noted within 2 days. Pain relief persisted in 75% of the survivors at 6 months.[33] Another series reported better results in solid tumor metastases than for myeloma.[27] Several different histologic types have been described, including kidney, breast, thyroid, bladder, lung, hepatocellular carcinoma, pheochromocytoma, prostate, and hemangiopericytoma.[9] One report described the use of vertebroplasty in recurrent collapse after irradiation for Langerhans' cell vertebral histiocytosis.[35]

There has been little written about the use of kyphoplasty in metastatic disease to the spine. Balloon expansion may cause embolization of neoplastic tissue. This has not been documented, and its risk should not be functionally different from that of tumor displacement with high-pressure PMMA injection during vertebroplasty. Void creation, allowing a more viscous PMMA to be used, may limit extravasation through perforations of the vertebral cortex.

VBA may be tumoricidal. Some authors state that PMMA has no effect on local tumor necrosis.[32] However, free monomer cytotoxicity, or the heat of polymerization, may destroy neoplastic cells.[9] In one report a decrease in serum metanephrine levels was noted after vertebroplasty in pheochromocytoma patients.[9]

Ultimately, vertebroplasty and kyphoplasty may be used as an adjunct to other treatment modalities. VBA does not interfere with subsequent radiation therapy, and radiation therapy does not interfere with the mechanical properties of the PMMA.[36] Vertebroplasty has been shown to be effective as a salvage modality in patients with continued pain after x-ray therapy (XRT).[9] VBA may also be used as an adjunct in selected patients undergoing open decompression or stabilization. In general, these techniques are reserved for patients with disseminated disease.

Vertebral Hemangioma

Although vertebroplasty was first described for use in hemangiomas, these lesions have encompassed only a small part of the North American experience.[8] Given the prevalence of back pain, the main difficulty lies in identifying symptomatic hemangiomas. In autopsy studies, 12% of an unselected population was noted to have spinal hemangiomas.[37] Some authors have tried to identify factors associated with hemangioma aggressiveness

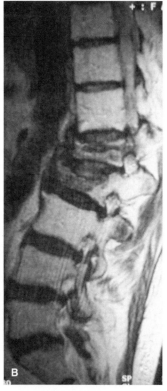

FIGURE 7–1 Six-month progression of deformity in a patient with prostate metastasis despite external-beam irradiation of the spine. This patient had immediate and sustained pain relief after kyphoplasty.

TABLE 7–2 Characteristics of Symptomatic Hemangiomas in the Spine

Location between T3 and T9
Involvement of the entire body
Extension to the neural arch
An expanded cortex with indistinct margins
An irregular honeycomb pattern
Soft tissue mass
Low fat content on MRI or CT

and hence clinical symptoms (Table **7–2**).[37,38] Results in limited series suggest greater than 90% pain relief.[37,39]

Bone Fragility

Other patient populations with fragile bone and a propensity for low-energy compression fractures may also benefit from VBA procedures. Our limited experience with osteogenesis imperfecta suggests that the indications and results are similar to those noted in older patients with osteoporosis.

■ Precautions/Contraindications

Several factors limit the application of VBA techniques despite a painful mechanical insufficiency of the anterior column of the spine (Table **7–3**). At this time, infection represents an absolute contraindication. Osteomyelitis of the target vertebral body or diskitis of the disk spaces above or below the intended level carries a significant risk of PMMA seeding. Certain technical and medical factors increase the procedural risk and,

TABLE 7–3 Precautions and Contraindications to VBA

Neurologic symptoms
Young patients
Pregnancy
High-velocity fractures
Fractured pedicles or facets
Burst fracture with retropulsed bone
Medical issues
Allergy to devices
Allergy to contrast medium
Bleeding disorders
Severe cardiopulmonary difficulties
Technically not feasible
Vertebra plana
Multiple painful vertebral bodies
Level above T5
Neoplasm
Osteoblastic metastasis
Patients with significant long-term survivability
Primary spinal neoplasm
Severe cortical destruction
Local spinal infection

therefore, represent precautions. Kyphoplasty or vertebroplasty may be offered in these cases only after careful risk-benefit analysis.

Vertebra Plana

Vertebra plana may make it difficult to safely insert the kyphoplasty instruments or a large-gauge vertebroplasty needle into the vertebral body. In the literature, minimal remaining vertebral height percentages are often quoted. Some authors do not attempt vertebroplasty if the target level is less than one third its normal height.[9,32,40] On the other hand, global percentages alone may not accurately reflect suitability. For example, safe canalization of a 50% collapsed thoracic vertebra may be impossible whereas larger lumbar vertebrae may be accessible with even 75% height loss.[25] In that the greatest height loss is in the center of the vertebral body, successful access to fractures with greater than 70% height loss can be achieved with a posterolateral (in the lumbar) or lateral extrapedicular approach.[41] In our experience, preoperative planning is more helpful than set numerical limits. We employ sagittally reconstructed computed tomography (CT) or parasagittal magnetic resonance imaging (MRI) to assess trajectory and determine if a safe approach is available.

With kyphoplasty, the inflatable tamps may be gradually advanced and inflated, thereby expanding the access tract to the anterior portions of the vertebral body (Fig. **7–2**). If only limited reduction is possible, smaller gauge Jamshidi needles and a vertebroplasty technique should be substituted. In acute fractures, a partial, positional reduction may be obtained through lordotic operative positioning (Fig. **7–3**).

Jensen and Dion[10] suggest that patients with >90% height loss do not respond well to vertebroplasty. Similarly, in O'Brien et al's[41] technical report, only four of six patients with greater than 70% height loss had pain relief.

Posterior Cortical Disruption and Pedicular Involvement

Incompetence of the posterior cortex in patients suffering low-energy pathologic fractures of the vertebral body is common. Although this disruption increases the risk of cement extrusion, it is not a direct contraindication to VBA. Successful vertebroplasty has been reported in cancer patients with significant bone loss of the posterior vertebral body.[9]

Some authors limit posterior retropulsion to a set proportion of canal diameter. Jensen and Dion,[10] for example, recommend vertebroplasty only when the retropulsed fragment is less than 20% of the canal

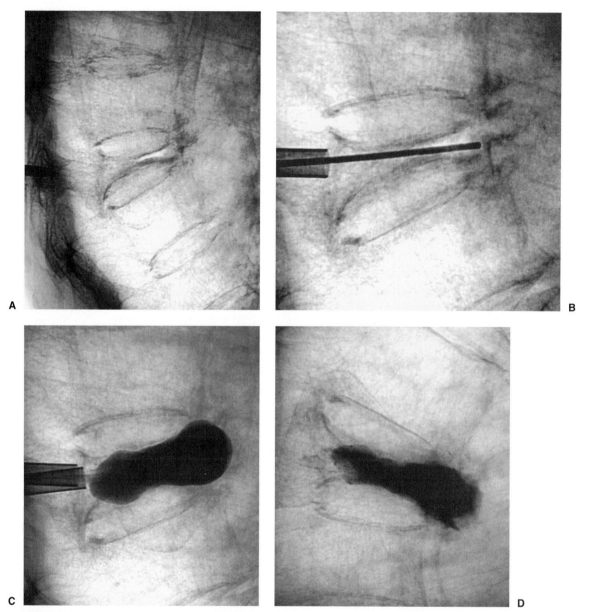

FIGURE 7–2 Serial balloon inflation and advancement was used to treat this patient with painful vertebra plana. Computed tomography (CT) measurements of vertebral height demonstrated a doubling of anterior and middle height measures. The patient reported 50% pain relief of axial pain with substantial improvement in thoracic radicular pain.

diameter. Certainly, severe posterior cortical disruption increases the risk and complexity of this procedure and should not be attempted early in a surgeon's experience with VBA. Evidence of neurologic compromise must be sought prior to the procedure and, if appropriate, decompression planned.

If the neoplasm or fracture has violated the pedicle, that pedicle should not be used for access to the vertebral centrum. This is particularly true in high-energy fractures. In the lumbar spine, a posterolateral extrapedicular approach may be substituted for the transpedicular approach if tumor is involving the pedicle.[9] An extrapedicular approach, between the rib head and pedicle, can be employed in the thoracic spine.

Upper Thoracic Levels

With the large-gauge instrumentation presently available, kyphoplasty is effectively limited to vertebral levels T5 and below. Vertebroplasty, on the other hand, may take advantage of smaller needles and has been successfully performed up to T2. However, imaging of the upper thoracic spine is challenging. Anteroposterior (AP) fluoroscopy is limited by the great vessels and the cardiac silhouette. Lateral fluoroscopy is limited by

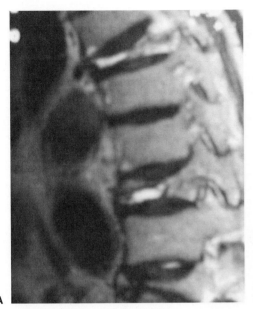
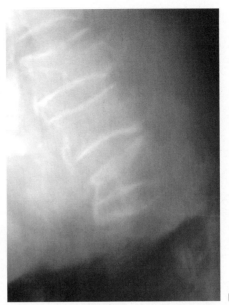

FIGURE 7–3 (A) Parasagittal T2 magnetic resonance imaging (MRI) suggesting major collapse and warning of technical difficulty in safe percutaneous device placement. **(B)** Scout lateral with patient prone with lordosing chest and pelvis roll. Fractures have partially reduced and instrumentation may be safely inserted.

superimposition of the shoulders. A CT-guided technique may provide better visualization of these challenging levels.[42] Upper thoracic fractures should be attempted only after significant practice in a cadaver laboratory and demonstrated competence with lower vertebral segments.

Multiple Painful Vertebral Bodies

Most patients present with focal pain originating at one or two segments. Others have diffuse pain throughout the spine. In that accurate identification of the pain generator is difficult, these patients are typically not good candidates for vertebroplasty or kyphoplasty.[10] However, if MRI or bone scan findings support multiple, unhealed fractures, multilevel VBA may be considered. In our experience, multiple myeloma patients have been the most responsive to multilevel VBA augmentation (Fig. 7–4).

Important considerations in these circumstances include the toxicity of large amounts of PMMA to be injected at multiple levels. If the procedure is to be performed with local anesthetic only, many patients will not tolerate lengthy periods in the prone position. Also, operator eye strain may compromise technique after two successive levels. On the other hand, if no general anesthesia is required, there is little risk in return for subsequent levels.

Prophylactic VBA has been described and remains controversial.[21,25]

■ Medical Issues

Coagulopathy is a common comorbidity in elderly patients with osteoporosis or in those with disseminated cancer. Osteoporotic or neoplastic bone is often quite vascular. Although PMMA will autoembolize the segment, cortical breaches may result in epidural hematoma. Prothrombin time (PT), partial thromboplastin time (PTT), and platelet counts should be assessed preoperatively in these patients. In our practice, intravenous (IV) heparin is stopped prior to VBA and the procedure is performed when the PTT has normalized. In patients on Coumadin, medication is suspended until the INR is less than 1.5. We resume these agents a few days after the procedure.

Many patients with painful pathologic compression fractures have coexistent, severe cardiopulmonary problems. Due to breathing difficulties, they may not be able to tolerate prone positioning for the duration of the procedure. Positioning is assessed in the preoperative evaluation. The benefits of airway control are balanced against the risks of general anesthesia in this patient population. Although general anesthesia may precipitate functional decline in patients with severe pulmonary insufficiency,[9] these patients must be able to tolerate emergent operative decompression should PMMA extravasation be noted.

When VBA is performed under local anesthesia, PMMA embolism may be detected immediately, by the onset of chest pain.[43] Similarly, complaints of radiating

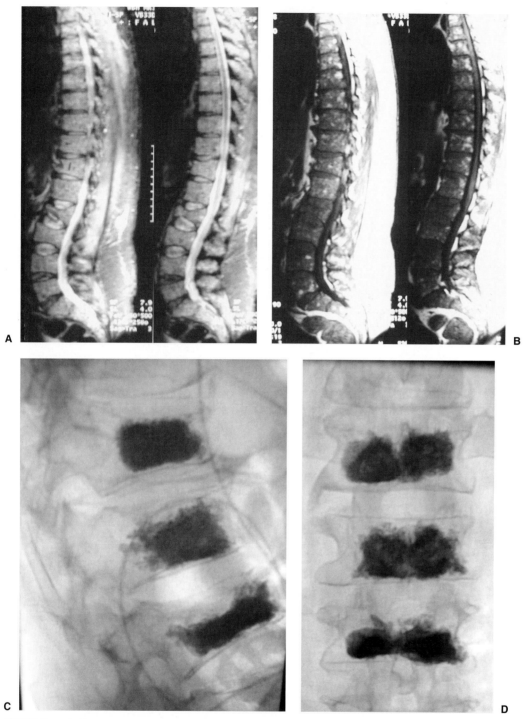

FIGURE 7–4 Multiple myeloma patient with multiple painful compression fractures for which he was on bed rest with IV narcotics. At 6-month follow-up from kyphoplasty, he is pain free and walking.

pain into the legs or anterior body wall suggest instrument or PMMA impingement of exiting nerves.

In patients with neurologic symptoms, any area of neurologic compression must be identified prior to consideration of VBA. If percutaneous vertebroplasty or kyphoplasty is performed, the risk of adverse outcomes with even small amounts of cement extravasation is increased.

Depending on its source and severity, open decompression with adjunctive VBA may be preferable.[44]

Neoplasm

Kyphoplasty and vertebroplasty are indicated in certain subtypes of painful pathologic compression fractures.

Typically, VBA is reserved for those patients with disseminated disease. In patients with primary spinal malignancy or isolated disease and long anticipated survival (at least 6 months), open surgical extirpation of the tumor should be considered. The role of VBA in benign primary tumors of the spine remains to be defined.

Fractures in vertebrae containing osteoblastic metastasis (such as many prostate metastases), are uncommon. Addition of PMMA to the vertebral body is not likely to benefit the patient. Further, radiation and chemotherapy should be considered over VBA in patients with highly radiosensitive lesions and little mechanical compromise of the vertebral body. Patients with significant soft tissue extension beyond the affected vertebral body may get limited pain relief from kyphoplasty or vertebroplasty.[9]

There are additional, technical challenges when treating a patient with a spinal column neoplasm. Venous leaks of PMMA are thought more likely to occur with vascular lesions, such as metastases of thyroid cancer, renal carcinoma, or vertebral angiomas.[43] In this setting, a more viscous PMMA should be applied to only one to two levels per session. In some cases, an epidurogram prior to PMMA injection may be useful in directing subsequent instrumentation away from large sinusoids. We have not employed preprocedural embolization.

■ Clinical Evaluation

The single most important factor in patient selection for vertebroplasty or kyphoplasty is accurate determination of the pain generator. There are multiple possible causes of spine pain. Therefore, the clinical evaluation must be rigorous. Complete history, physical examination, and laboratory and imaging evaluations are undertaken prior to reaching conclusions about the appropriateness of VBA. The particular goals of patient evaluation are:

1. Accurate identification of the painful segment(s)
2. Delineation of symptomatic and functional impact
3. Exclusion of confounding or technical variables

■ History

A complete history is obtained. Particular attention is directed toward several key elements (Table 7–4). First, the treating physician must understand the mechanism of injury. Patients with pathologic compression fractures often describe minimal or no trauma prior to the onset of pain.

Symptom progression and severity should be noted. To understand the impact of the fracture, a symptom

TABLE 7–4 Elements in the History

Mechanism
Type of pain
Time course of symptoms
Radiation of pain
Review of systems
Previous fractures

diary including pain medication usage and functional limitations may be useful in some patients. Typical osteoporotic compression fracture symptoms improve over 4 to 6 weeks.[14] Failure to improve after this time merits more intensive evaluation.

The nature and location of the pain focus the subsequent exam and help predict success with VBA. Patients describing good to excellent relief of their preoperative symptoms after vertebroplasty or kyphoplasty most often have a focal, intense, deep pain in one or more areas of the midline of the spine before the procedure.[10] Those with diffuse pain or pain localized in the paravertebral musculature report little improvement after VBA.

Precipitating and palliating factors should be sought. Mechanical loading should increase the pain severity. Pain that is constant in intensity does not respond as well to VBA, as does pain that is relieved during recumbency.

Patients should describe any radiation of their pain. Thoracic radiation is not uncommon.[21] Bone fragments or foraminal stenosis from vertebral height loss may contribute to a thoracic radiculopathy. However, if radiculopathy is a major portion of the complaint, VBA should be considered only as a secondary treatment modality after steroid injection or other direct treatment of the nerve root irritation. In some settings kyphoplasty reduction of the vertebral body compression may relieve foraminal stenosis (Fig. 7–2).

Historical evidence of myelopathy is sought as well. Gait difficulties, clumsiness, weakness or sensory changes, electric shock sensations (Lhermitte's phenomenon), or bowel and bladder complaints are significant. Spinal cord symptoms are uncommon. Myelopathy may result from large posterior bone fragments or spinal cord impingement over kyphotic spinal segments. Myelopathy is decidedly more common in patients with vertebral metastases.[27]

The review of symptoms in the osteoporotic fracture group should include markers for inflammatory or neoplastic disease such as night pain, fevers, chills, and unusual weight loss.

Past medical history review includes treatment of underlying osteoporosis; history of cancer, tuberculosis, or systemic infection; and previous fractures of the axial or appendicular skeleton. In patients with previous vertebral compression fractures, effectiveness of attempted treatment, time course to healing, and days of bed rest are useful in predicting future treatment response.

TABLE 7–5 Elements of the Physical Examination

General condition
Gait
Spinal balance
Spinal vs. diffuse tenderness
Rib exam
Neurologic exam

TABLE 7–7 Fractures Less Likely to Improve with Standard Medical Management

Fractures at the thoracolumbar junction (T11-L2)
Burst fracture
Wedge compression fractures with >30 degrees of sagittal angulation
Vacuum shadow in fractured body (ischemic necrosis of bone)
Progressive collapse on radiographic follow-up

Physical Exam

A brief general physical examination and a detailed evaluation of the spine and neurologic system are important aspects of patient selection for kyphoplasty or vertebroplasty (Table 7–5). On first encounter several aspects of the patient's general physical condition may be assessed, including breathing and body habitus (which may limit effective bracing). The patient's gait is evaluated, and evidence of abdominal and rib tenderness sought. Coexisting, or iatrogenic, rib fractures are common in the osteoporotic patient population undergoing VBA.

The spine exam includes assessment of spinal balance (kyphosis) and tenderness. Tenderness should be midline and focal to one or several spinous processes. Evidence of polymyalgia or diffuse or superficial tenderness should discourage invasive therapy. Similarly, patients with significant facet pain, if it can be determined, may not benefit from VBA.

Neurologic examination includes a search for thoracic radiculopathy by dermatomal sensory examination. Strength, sensation, and vascular status are assessed in the extremities. Deep tendon and pathologic reflex tests should be performed.

Finally, the patient's ability to tolerate prone positioning in terms of discomfort and breathing is tested.

Imaging

Imaging remains a cornerstone of patient selection for kyphoplasty and vertebroplasty (Table 7–6). Radiographs, MRI, and occasionally scintigraphy confirm the diagnosis and add valuable information as to the technical practicality of VBA. Imaging findings may predict which fractures will respond to nonoperative care (Table 7–7).

Plain Radiography

Typical fractures in the thoracic spine and thoracolumbar junction have a wedge appearance, due to anterior

TABLE 7–6 Goals of Imaging

Extent of vertebral collapse
Location and extent of lytic process
Visibility and degree of involvement of the pedicles
Presence of cortical destruction or fracture
Presence of epidural or foraminal stenosis
Age or acuity of the fracture

column loading and kyphotic angulation. In the lumbar spine, central end-plate cupping of lordotic lumbar bodies is more common.[45] In one large epidemiologic study, all fracture types were found to be painful.[45]

Plain radiographs alone are not precise in determining fracture age. Comparison films, or previous lateral chest radiographs, may be helpful for thoracic fractures. Sclerosis alone is problematic because the additional radiopacity may represent bone healing, or merely compressed trabeculae.

Spot lateral films are helpful, particularly at the thoracolumbar junction where lung shadows can make careful evaluation of a compressed, osteoporotic, vertebra difficult. Evidence of posterior cortical compromise is also sought. Widened pedicles may be seen on the AP films. On lateral radiographs, buckling of the posterior cortex or greater than 50% posterior cortical height loss implies canal compromise. Long films are also helpful as a means of assessing and following sagittal spinal balance.

Other pathology may be manifest on plain radiographs. End-plate erosion and disk space loss may signal osteomyelitis. Unilateral absence of the pedicle on the AP (winking owl sign) or fractures above T6 are more likely to represent neoplasm.[14]

Plain radiographs give an excellent approximation of the technical feasibility of the procedure. If pedicles cannot be visualized on multiple attempts at AP radiographs, safe access to that segment in the operating room or imaging suite may be very difficult or impossible. As mentioned above, certain cases of significant height loss may also restrict access to that segment.

Nonoperatively managed patients warrant close radiographic follow-up. Further collapse, progress, or excessive kyphosis, even if relatively asymptomatic, may warrant VBA.

Advanced Imaging

Several advanced imaging modalities allow for further assessment of the fracture in question and the patient, in general (Table 7–8).

Dual-energy x-ray absorptiometry (DEXA) reflects a useful means of measuring spinal bone mineral content with a low dose of radiation to the patient. In that DEXA confers precision within 1 to 2% at the spine and 3 to 4% at the femur, it is the modality of choice for quantification of osteoporosis. DEXA values are falsely increased

TABLE 7–8 Imaging Features Suggestive of Malignancy

Location between T3 and T9
Involvement of the entire body
Extension to the neural arch
An expanded cortex with indistinct margins
An irregular honeycomb pattern
Soft tissue mass
Low-fat content on MRI or CT

with scoliosis, compression fractures, significant degenerative joint disease, and in those with extraosseous calcification and vascular disease.

MRI is the modality of choice for close assessment of both fracture architecture and acuity. Acute fractures contain bands of edema, which are reflected by increased signal on T2 or short-time inversion recovery (STIR) sequences. STIR (TR/TE 4000/60, inversion time 150 msec), with 5-mm sections in the sagittal plane sequences, identifies physiologically active fractures that respond well to VBA.[46] On T1-weighted images, an acute or unhealed fracture demonstrates a decreased signal. In osteoporotic fractures the signal changes with time, representing healing. In the first 4 months the signal is low on T1 and high T2 with a band pattern that involves a band either across the portion of the vertebral body whose end plate is fractured or across the end body (R1) (Fig. 7–5). After 6 months the signal tends to normalize.

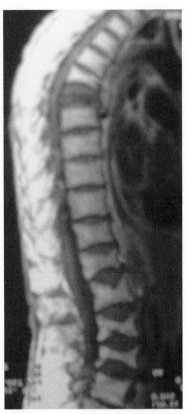

FIGURE 7–6 T1-weighted MRI parasagittal image of T7 acute compression fracture. Note previous, healed fractures at L1-L4 with restoration of normal marrow signal.

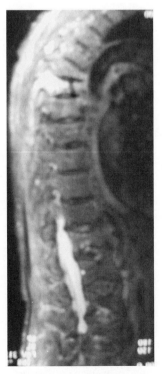

FIGURE 7–5 STIR sequence parasagittal MRI image of acute T7 compression fracture.

Occasionally, despite many months, marrow signal patterns continue to appear acute. MRI signal changes disappear several months before normalization of an increase of technetium uptake in bone scans (Fig. 7–6) (R1).

There is some evidence to suggest that painful fractures more than 1 year old may not respond to the VBA.[10] In our experience, however, pain response is more closely related to the severity of the signal change on the MRI, particularly a large, intense T2 signal band below the fracture, than the chronicity of the fracture in temporal terms.

Differentiating osteoporotic compression fractures from those caused by metastases is difficult. In metastatic disease, T1 signal is decreased. T2 signal is usually increased, either in the whole vertebral body or in a patchy distribution within it (R1). Signal differences were found in one study to be sensitive, but not specific in the differentiation of neoplastic as opposed to osteoporotic compression fracture.[47]

Soft tissue extension signals neoplasm. Also, with metastases the signal change is more likely to extend into the pedicle and posterior arch than with osteoporotic fractures. These patients are more likely to demonstrate a diffuse posterior cortical wall bulge (R1). In osteoporotic

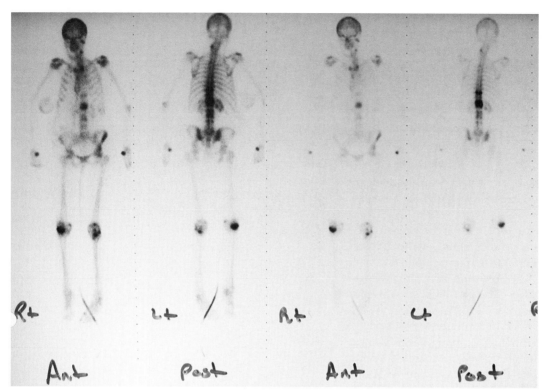

FIGURE 7–7 Technetium bone scan demonstrating increased uptake at T11 and L1 4 months after the onset of thoracolumbar junction spine pain after lifting a potted plant.

fractures, a recession of one of the corners of the vertebral body may be noted (R1). In one study, MRI had a 92% specificity between malignant and benign compression fractures and was more sensitive than bone scan for this purpose (R1). The addition of gadolinium does not increase MRI's sensitivity, or specificity, in differentiating these lesions.[47]

CT scans offer high bone and soft tissue contrast. This contrast is useful in delineating cortical compromise. CT is also the modality of choice to demonstrate suspected posterior element or pedicle fractures. In the typical patient, however, MRI is preferred. When MRI is not available, CT and technetium scintigraphy in combination are appropriate substitutes.

A technetium bone scan demonstrates increased uptake in areas of bone formation (Fig. **7–7**). Aggressively destructive lesions with little new bone formation (such as multiple myeloma, plasmacytoma, and metastases of certain histologic types) may not appear on bone scan. When these vertebral bodies succumb to pathologic fracture, however, the bone scan usually becomes positive. One study found increased uptake on bone scan highly predictive for successful outcome from vertebroplasty.[48]

Several different recommendations have been made with regard to the timing of imaging in patients with pathologic compression fractures. In patients with changing symptoms, old MRI and bone scan data may no longer be accurate. Some authors recommend a CT within 3 days of the procedure.[27,32] If this is not feasible, close comparison of scout films with previously obtained studies is warranted. Several of our patients have had new, interval fractures between office evaluation and the procedure date.

■ Patient Selection and Decision Making

Careful patient evaluation identifies those fractures most amenable to VBA. Close concordance of the history, examination, and imaging studies helps predict success in a high percentage of patients. Unfortunately, the vast majority of papers discussing vertebroplasty describe little of the historical and physical examination data incorporated into patient selection.[8,21,32,37,38,40] In one study, pain of greater than 1 month's duration was an excluding factor, and all fractures with positive signal change on MRI or scintigraphy were treated.[46] Based on the natural history of compression fractures and the significant percentage of patients referred for VBA with sciatica or other pain, the radiologist or other non–spine care clinician should be cautious in the selection of patients for this procedure.[45]

Once an acute compression fracture has been diagnosed, several nonsurgical modalities are available. A multidisciplinary approach is often helpful.[25] In osteoporosis patients, appropriate assessment of bone mineral density followed by management of the underlying osteoporosis is instituted in all patients. Nasal calcitonin and bisphosphonates have been shown to decrease the pain associated with compression fracture and to improve function.[50] In patients with fractures due to malignancy, consultation with the oncology team improves understanding of the degree of dissemination and the patient's prognosis. Radiation or chemotherapy in conjunction with, or instead of, VBA should always be considered.

A short period of relative rest is recommended, as are narcotic pain medications. The pain usually lasts 4 to 6 weeks but can often continue for months. Pain medications should be continued until the patient can bear weight comfortably. In the elderly, use of narcotics may be associated with as many functional problems as the underlying fracture itself. The effectiveness of these medications in alleviating pain and restoring function must be compared with side effects, including mental status changes, constipation, and increased risk of falling.

Orthotics may allow early ambulation with decreased pain in selected patients. Braces should be easy to fit and wear to improve compliance. Typically, a lightweight extension brace such as a tri-pad Jewett or Cash brace is selected.[3] These braces allow axial loading and leave the chest and torso free. For lumbar-level fractures, a corset may be recommended. Brace-wear is continued until the patient is comfortable and no progression of deformity is noted on serial radiographs.

Braces are not appropriate for all patients, however. Many patients with obesity or severe deformity are simply not effectively braced. Some authors report low brace compliance, citing shoulder problems and other mechanical interference to donning and doffing the brace.[49] Brace dependence is to be avoided. After the fracture has begun to heal, physical therapy to improve posture, strength, and range of motion is indicated.

Despite appropriate use of these nonoperative modalities, over 200,000 compression fractures per year are refractory to narcotics. In these patients, long-term immobility and its secondary effects are noted in episodes that can last from weeks to months. Intractable pain leads to 150,000 hospital admissions per year.

The timing of operative intervention is an important element in the kyphoplasty decision-making process.

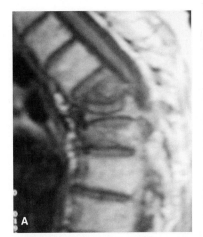
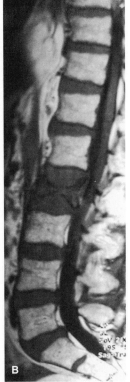

FIGURE 7–8 (A) Parasagittal MRI of multiple thoracic fractures bearing many stigmata mitigating for early treatment, including a bursting pattern and local kyphosis >30 degrees. (B) Stigmata of fracture in which a period of nonoperative treatment is indicated prior to vertebral body augmentation (VBA). One level is involved, there is no retropulsion, and overall spinal alignment is maintained.

Arguments in favor of early stabilization include minimization of subsequent deformity and its effects on breathing and appetite, minimization of narcotic dependence and side effects, and the immediate restoration of patient function and independence. Delayed treatment may result in the avoidance of operative risks altogether due to the high rate of spontaneous healing and symptom regression.

Nonoperative treatment intervals should usually last at least 3 to 6 weeks.[10,24] For those whose pain continues after this interval, kyphoplasty can be considered. Early kyphoplasty can be offered to those at significant risk for functional decline or decubiti. Early kyphoplasty is also suggested for those unable to ambulate despite several days of appropriate pharmacologic pain management. Those unable to tolerate bracing or an effective narcotic regimen may benefit from earlier intervention (Fig. 7–8). Finally, early kyphoplasty may be suggested if serial collapse of the fracture is noted on radiographic follow-up.

REFERENCES

1. Silverman SL. The clinical consequences of vertebral compression fracture. Bone 1992;13(suppl 2):S27–S31
2. Schachar NS. An update on the nonoperative treatment of patients with metastatic bone disease. Clin Orthop 2001;382:75–81
3. Rapado A. General management of vertebral fractures. Bone 1996;18:191S–196S
4. Bostrom MP, Lane JM. Future directions: augmentation of osteoporotic vertebral bodies. Spine 1997;22(24 suppl):38S–42S. Erratum in: Spine 1998;23(17):1922
5. Belkoff SM, Mathis JM, Erbe EM, Fenton DC. Biomechanical evaluation of a new bone cement for use in vertebroplasty. Spine 2000;25:1061–1064
6. Dean JR, Ison KT, Gishen P. The strengthening effect of percutaneous vertebroplasty. Clin Radiol 2000;55:471–476
7. Belkoff SM, Mathis JM, Fenton DC, Scribner RM, Reiley ME, Talmadge K. An ex vivo biomechanical evaluation of an inflatable bone tamp used in the treatment of compression fracture. Spine 2001;26:151–156
8. Deramond H, Depriester C, Galibert P, Le Gars D. Percutaneous vertebroplasty with polymethylmethacrylate: technique, indications, and results. Radiol Clin North Am 1998;36:533–546
9. Weill A, Chiras J, Simon JM, Rose M, Sola-Martinez T, Enkaoua E. Spinal metastases: indications for and results of percutaneous injection of an acrylic surgical cement. Radiology 1996;199:241–247
10. Jensen ME, Dion JE. Percutaneous vertebroplasty in the treatment of osteoporotic compression fractures. Neuroimaging Clin North Am 2000;10:547–568
11. Murphy KJ, Deramond H. Percutaneous vertebroplasty in benign and malignant disease. Neuroimaging Clin North Am 2000;10:535–545
12. Gold DT. The clinical impact of vertebral fractures: quality of life in women with osteoporosis. Bone 1996;18:185S–189S
13. Melton LJ III. Epidemiology of vertebral fractures in women. Am J Epidemiol 1989;129:1000–1011
14. Tamayo-Orozco J, Arzac-Palumbo P, Peon-Vidales H, Mota-Bolfeta R, Fuentes F. Vertebral fractures associated with osteoporosis: patient management. Am J Med 1997;103:44S–48S
15. Nevitt MC, Ettinger B, Black DM, et al. The association of radiographically detected vertebral fractures with back pain and function: a prospective study. Ann Intern Med 1998;128:793–800
16. Miller PD. New guidelines for the prevention and treatment of osteoporosis. Adv Intern Med 1999;44:175–207
17. Cauley JA, Seeley DG, Ensrud K, Ettinger B, Black D, Cummings SR. Estrogen replacement therapy and fractures in older women. Study of Osteoporotic Fractures Research Group. Ann Intern Med 1995;122:9–16
18. Ettinger B, Black DM, Mitlak BH, et al, and the Multiple Outcomes of Raloxifene Evaluation (MORE) Investigators. Reduction of vertebral fracture risk in postmenopausal women with osteoporosis treated with raloxifene: results from a 3-year randomized clinical trial. JAMA 1999;282:637–645
19. Liberman UA, Weiss SR, Broll J, et al. Effect of oral alendronate on bone mineral density and the incidence of fractures in postmenopausal osteoporosis. The Alendronate Phase III Osteoporosis Treatment Study Group. N Engl J Med 1995;333:1437–1443
20. Pal B, Morris J, Muddu B. The management of osteoporosis-related fractures: a survey of orthopaedic surgeons' practice. Clin Exp Rheumatol 1998;16:61–62
21. Jensen ME, Evans AJ, Mathis JM, et al. Percutaneous polymethylmethacrylate vertebroplasty in the treatment of osteoporotic vertebral body compression fractures: technical aspects. AJNR Am J Neuroradiol 1997;18:1897–1904
22. Wasnich RD. Vertebral fracture epidemiology. Bone 1996;18 (3 suppl):179S–183S
23. Martin JB, Jean B, Sugui K, et al. Vertebroplasty: clinical experience and follow-up results. Bone 1999;25:11S–15S
24. Grados F, Depriester C, Cayrolle G, Hardy N, Deramond H, Fardellone P. Long-term observations of vertebral osteoporotic fractures treated by percutaneous vertebroplasty. Rheumatology (Oxf) 2000;39:1410–1414
25. Barr JD, Barr MS, Lemley TJ, McCann RM. Percutaneous vertebroplasty for pain relief and spinal stabilization. Spine 2000;25:923–928
26. Cortet B, Cotten A, Boutry N, et al. Percutaneous vertebroplasty in the treatment of osteoporotic vertebral compression fractures: an open prospective study. J Rheumatol 1999;26:2222–2228
27. Cotten A, Dewatre F, Cortet B, et al. Percutaneous vertebroplasty for osteolytic metastases and myeloma: effects of the percentage of lesion filling and the leakage of methyl methacrylate at clinical follow-up. Radiology 1996;200:525–530
28. Schachar NS. An update on the nonoperative treatment of patients with metastatic bone disease. Clin Orthop 2001; 382:75–81
29. Shepard S. Radiotherapy and the management of metastatic bone pain. Clin Radiol 1988;39:547–550
30. Gilbert HA, Kagan AR, Nussbaum H, et al. Evaluation of radiation therapy for bone metastases: pain relief and quality of life. AJR Am J Roentgenol 1977;129:1095–1096
31. Salazar OM, Rubin P, Hendrickson FR, et al. Single-dose half-body irradiation for palliation of multiple bone metastases from solid tumors. Cancer 1986;58:29–36
32. Cotten A, Boutry N, Cortet B, et al. Percutaneous vertebroplasty: state of the art. Radiographics 1998;18(2):311–320; discussion 320–323
33. Cortet B, Cotten A, Boutry N, et al. Percutaneous vertebroplasty in patients with osteolytic metastases or multiple myeloma. Rev Rhum Engl Ed 1997;64:177–183
34. Lafforgue P, Bayle O, Massonnat J, et al. L'IRM au cours des tassements vertebraux osteoporotiques et metastatiques: a propos de soixante cas. Ann Radiol (Paris) 1991;34:157–166
35. Cardon T, Hachulla E, Flipo RM, et al. Percutaneous vertebroplasty with acrylic cement in the treatment of a Langerhans' cell vertebral histiocytosis. Clin Rheumatol 1994;13:518–521
36. Murray JA, Bruels MC, Lindberg R. Irradiation of polymethylmethacrylate. J Bone Joint Surg 1974;56-A:311–312
37. Ide C, Gangi A, Rimmelin A, et al. Vertebral haemangiomas with spinal cord compression: the place of preoperative percutaneous vertebroplasty with methyl methacrylate. Neuroradiology 1996;38:585–589
38. Laredo JD, Assouline E, Gelbert F, Wybier M, Merland JJ, Tubiana JM. Vertebral hemangiomas: fat content as a sign of aggressiveness. Radiology 1990;177:467–472
39. Deramond H, Daasson R, Galibert P. Percutaneous vertebroplasty with acrylic cement in the treatment of aggressive spinal angiomas. Rachis 1989;1:143–153
40. Mathis JM, Petri M, Naff N. Percutaneous vertebroplasty treatment of steroid induced osteoporotic compression fractures. Arthritis Rheum 1998;41:171–175
41. O'Brien JP, Sims JT, Evans AJ. Vertebroplasty in patients with severe vertebral compression fractures: a technical report. AJNR Am J Neuroradiol 2000;21:1555–1558
42. Gangi A, Kastler BA, Dietemann JL. Percutaneous vertebroplasty guided by a combination of CT and fluoroscopy. AJNR Am J Neuroradiol 1994;15:83–86
43. Padovani B, Kasriel O, Brunner P, Peretti-Viton P. Pulmonary embolism caused by acrylic cement: a rare complication of percutaneous vertebroplasty. AJNR Am J Neuroradiol 1999;20:375–377
44. Cortet B, Cotten A, Deprez X, et al. ([Value of vertebroplasty combined with surgical decompression in the treatment of aggressive spinal angioma: apropos of three cases]) Interet de la vertebroplastie couplee a une decompression chirurgicale dans le traitement

des angiomes vertebraux agressifs: a propos de trois cas. Rev Rhum Ed Fr 1994;61:16–22

45. Ismail AA, Cooper C, Felsenburg D, et al. Number and type of vertebral deformities: epidemiological characteristics and relation to back pain and height loss. Osteoporos Int 1999;9: 206–213

46. Cyteval C, Sarrabere MP, Roux JO, et al. Acute osteoporotic vertebral collapse: open study on percutaneous injection of acrylic surgical cement in 20 patients. AJR Am J Roentgenol 1999;173: 1685–1690

47. Rupp RE, Ebraheim NA, Coombs RJ. Magnetic resonance imaging differentiation of compression spine fractures or vertebral lesions caused by osteoporosis or tumor. Spine 1995;20(23):2499–2503; discussion 2504

48. Maynard AS, Jensen ME, Schweickert PA, Marx WF, Short JG, Kallmes DF. Value of bone scan imaging in predicting pain relief from percutaneous vertebroplasty in osteoporotic vertebral fractures. AJNR Am J Neuroradiol 2000;21:1807–1812

49. Einhorn TA. Vertebroplasty: an opportunity to do something really good for patients. Spine 2000;25:1051–1052

50. Nevitt MC, Thompson DE, Black DM, et al. Effect of alendronate on limited-activity days and bed-disability days caused by back pain in postmenopausal women with existing vertebral fractures. Arch Intern Med 2000;160:77–85

8

Technique and Pitfalls of Kyphoplasty

MARK A. REILEY

Objectives: On completion of this chapter, the reader should be able to (1) describe the potential morbidity associated with vertebral compression fracture and (2) discuss selection criteria for vertebroplasty and kyphoplasty.

Accreditation: The American Association of Neurological Surgeons is accredited by the Accreditation Council for Continuing Medical Education to sponsor continuing medical education for physicians.

Credit: The American Association of Neurological Surgeons designates this continuing medical education activity for a maximum of 15 credits in Category I of the Physician's Recognition Award of the American Medical Association.

The Home Study Examination is online at www.aans.org/education/books/vertebro.asp

The National Osteoporosis Foundation estimates that over 100 million people worldwide, and nearly 30 million in the United States, are at risk to develop fragility fractures secondary to osteoporosis. In the United States there are an estimated 700,000 pathologic vertebral body compression fractures each year, of which over one third become chronically painful.[1,2] The majority of these fractures (~85%) are the result of primary osteoporosis, the remainder due to secondary osteoporosis or lytic spinal metastases. These compression fractures lead to progressive deformity and changes in spinal biomechanics and are believed to contribute to increased risk of further fracture. Whether the fracture is painful or not, the resultant spinal deformity impacts health, daily living, and medical costs, through loss of lung capacity, reduced mobility, chronic pain, loss of appetite, and clinical depression.[3–9] With each osteoporotic vertebral compression fracture, there is a 9% loss in forced vital capacity (with both thoracic and lumbar fractures), a 23% age-adjusted increase in mortality,[10] and a 5-year survival rate less than that for hip fractures.[11] Osteoporotic vertebral compression fractures are clearly a clinically significant health problem with continuously increasing economic and social issues. The National Osteoporosis Foundation predicts that the number of vertebral body compression fractures will double in the next 15 years, due to the aging population and our increasingly sedentary lifestyles.

Traditionally, vertebral body compression fractures were treated with medical and only rarely with surgical modalities. Unfortunately, the medical management of painful fractures (bed rest, hospitalization, narcotic analgesics, and bracing) does nothing to restore spinal alignment and may compound the problem. Due to its inherent risks, invasive nature, and the poor quality of osteoporotic bone, the surgical treatment of vertebral body compression fractures has been limited to cases where there is concurrent spinal instability or neurologic deficit.

In response to the limited results of medical and surgical modalities, to stabilize and strengthen the collapsed vertebral bodies, interventional neuroradiologists, first in France and now the United States, initiated transpedicular percutaneous bone cement injections.[12,13] Direct cement injection, known as vertebroplasty, has been shown to reduce or eliminate fracture pain.

Vertebroplasty, however, does not address the spinal deformity. Also, this technique requires a high-pressure cement injection using low-viscosity cement, thus increasing the risk of cement leaks through the fracture clefts or the venous sinuses.

Kyphoplasty is a more recent technique—the first procedure was performed in September 1998 by the author. It has several potential advantages. Kyphoplasty involves the extra- or transpedicular cannulation of the vertebral body, under fluoroscopic guidance, followed by insertion of an inflatable bone tamp. Once inflated, the tamp restores the vertebral body back toward its original height, while creating a cavity to be filled with bone cement (Fig. 8–1). The cement application is

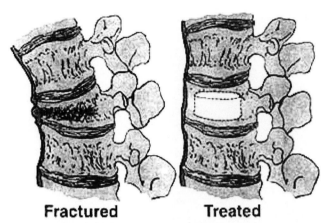

Fractured   Treated

FIGURE 8–1 Pre- and postkyphoplasty.

done under relatively low pressure and with cement that is far along in its polymerization phase in an attempt to reduce the risk of extravasation.

■ Indications

Kyphoplasty is indicated for progressive, painful osteoporotic or osteolytic vertebral body wedge compression fracture for both acute fractures, 1 to 2 weeks old, and chronic fractures. The percentage of height restoration is nearly 100% when compression fractures are treated early; that is, in the first 2 weeks (Fig. 8–2). After 2½ weeks fracture reduction is less predictable. For example, Fig. 8–3 shows three fractures above a three-level fusion. L2 and T12 compression fractures occurred 3 weeks prekyphoplasty, and L1 was of indeterminate age. T12 was elevated 14 mm; however, the L2 fracture was not reduced at all. However, on occasion an older compression fracture may be reducible with the bone balloon (Fig. 8–4).

Vertebroplasties, the free-hand injection of wet cement into vertebral body fractures, are not done for acute fractures because the risk of cement leakage into the spinal canal is considerable. Like any other fracture, the goals for compression fractures of the spine should be to restore stability and bony anatomic alignment, prevent deformity, and restore function as soon as safely possible. Like hip fracture surgery, the results are optimized with immediate operative intervention before muscle wasting and malnutrition become obstacles to the patient's recovery.

The contraindications to kyphoplasty include sepsis, prolonged bleeding times, and cardiopulmonary pathology (especially essential pulmonary hypertension and severe aortic stenosis), which would preclude the safe completion of the procedure under either conscious sedation or general anesthesia. Other relative contraindications include solid tumor spinal metastases, vertebral bodies with deficient posterior cortices, and neurologic signs or symptoms. Certain burst or vertebra plana fracture configurations (with the superior end plate depressed below the level of the pedicles) are technically difficult, and introduce the risk of segmental artery injury to the kyphoplasty procedure. The treatment of these fractures should be assessed on the merits of the case. In many cases their treatment should be avoided.

■ Preoperative Planning

For kyphoplasty the preoperative planning involves physical examination and radiologic evaluation. Radiographs, computed tomography (CT) scans, magnetic resonance imaging (MRI) scans, and nuclear medicine bone scans

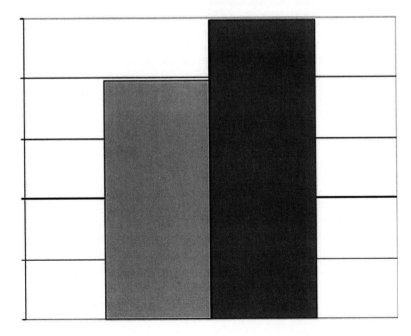

FIGURE 8–2 Height graph of 27 consecutive compression fractures treated within 2 weeks of injury. Ninety-nine percent of prefracture height is obtained if kyphoplasty is performed early.

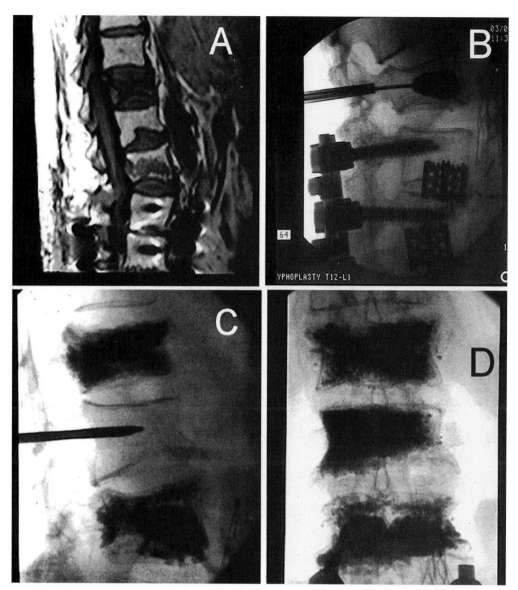

FIGURE 8–3 (A) Lateral magnetic resonance imaging (MRI) of three compression fractures. T12 is acute with hemorrhage present, L1 is of unknown age, L2 is acute with hemorrhage present, and L3 and L4 are part of a fusion. **(B)** Lateral, intraoperative C-arm image shows balloon as it expands in L2. **(C)** Lateral, intraoperative C-arm image after T12 and L2 have been cemented. Notice the height of T12 is increased ~14 mm and the height of L2 is unchanged, despite both fractures having acute hemorrhage and being the same age. An 11-gauge needle is in L1. **(D)** Anteroposterior (AP) intraoperative C-arm image of patient after three-level kyphoplasty. (Courtesy Dr. Mary Hume, Jackson Hole, Wyoming.)

are used to confirm the fracture and define the anatomy. The most reliable tools for diagnosing spinal compression fractures are the MRI, coupled with physical exam. Localized tenderness found on the spinous process on exam helps verify the level of fracture seen on MRI. Not infrequently the spinal palpation needs to be performed several times until pain is consistently found at one or a few levels. Plain radiographs are sufficient if comparison x-rays are less than 3 weeks old. The sagittal and axial CT and MRI scans are particularly important to plan the trajectory for any percutaneous spinal procedure.

■ Technique

Positioning and Anesthesia

The patient is positioned prone on the operating room table or in the radiology suite on a spinal frame or cushioned bolsters. If possible, positioning should promote extension of the thoracic and lumbar spine. The Kyphon tools, which are simple to use, are laid out on the back table (Figs. 8–5 and 8–6). Biplane fluoroscopy and single C-arm or double C-arm setups have all been used effectively for kyphoplasty. The radiologic

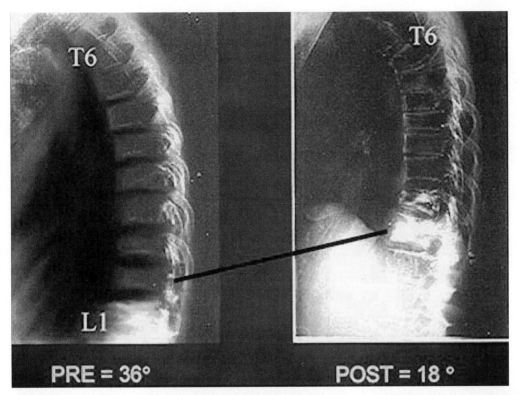

FIGURE 8–4 Lateral x-rays pre- and postkyphoplasty in an 89-year-old-woman with 9-month-old fractures. Preoperatively the patient had a kyphosis from T6 to L1 of 36 degrees, and postoperatively it measured 18 degrees.

equipment is positioned and tested to ensure all vertebral landmarks can be defined (pedicles, end plates, spinous processes, and vertebral body cortices). Precise alignment of bony landmarks on both anteroposterior (AP) and lateral views facilitates the kyphoplasty enormously (Fig. 8–7); even small amounts of improper x-ray alignment can make the procedure both more difficult and riskier (Fig. 8–8). Appropriate x-ray images may be difficult to obtain in some patients with severe osteo-

porosis, or more likely with poor C-arm equipment. In these cases, the procedure should not be performed.

Local anesthesia with intravenous conscious sedation, or general anesthesia may be used. If the patient has two or more fractures, it is more reasonable to perform the procedure under general anesthesia, or do multiple procedures at different sessions. Patients can tolerate a single-level procedure under local anesthetic with little discomfort, and in the medically ill patient, local

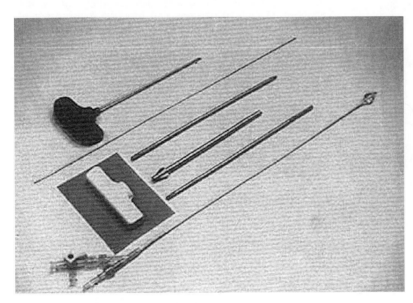

FIGURE 8–5 The tools used in the kyphoplasty procedure. From the top down: 11-gauge needle, guide pin, blunt obturator, cannula, drill bit, and Kyphon inflatable bone tamp.

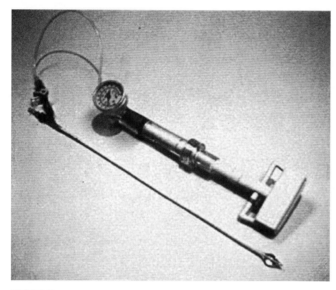

FIGURE 8–6 The inflatable bone tamp is attached to the insufflator.

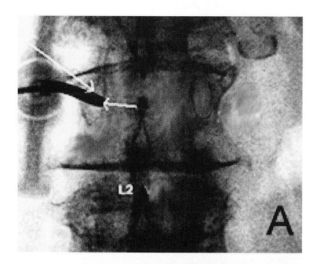

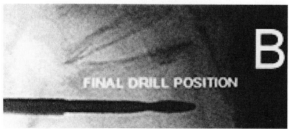

FIGURE 8–7 (A) An excellent AP C-arm view of L1. Note the pedicles are located in the top half of the vertebral body, nearly touching the shadow of the superior end plate. Also the spinous process is midline and the superior and inferior end plates are parallel. The 11-gauge needle is entering the left pedicle. **(B)** An excellent lateral C-arm view of L1. Note the pedicular shadows are overlapped and the superior and inferior end plates are parallel. The drill bit has been passed through the pedicle to within 3 mm of the anterior cortex, an appropriate stopping point for this tool.

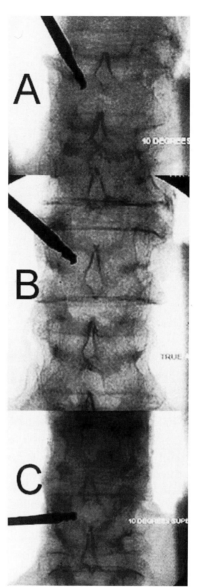

FIGURE 8–8 These three x-ray images demonstrate how variations of just 10 degrees can produce major problems with tool alignment. **(A)** The trajectory of the drill bit when the AP image is angled 10 degrees inferior to a straight AP. Note the drill bit appears to be angled too inferiorly. **(B)** A true AP of the same vertebral body and drill bit. In this view the angle of the drill bit is perfect, and no adjustment appears to be needed. **(C)** The same drill bit and vertebral body with the C-arm angled from 10 degrees superiorly and the drill bit appears to be aimed too superior in the vertebral body.

anesthesia may be preferable, but general anesthesia is usually the best for this procedure.

Transpedicular Approach

A transpedicular vertebral body cannulation can usually be used from T5 to L5 when performing a vertebroplasty. With kyphoplasty, the inflatable bone tamps need to be placed medially within the vertebral body, making transpedicular appropriate from T10 to L5. With correct placement, the pedicle guides the 11-gauge spinal

- The *en face* image
  may aid in tool
  placement

- Orient C-arm 10–20
  degrees oblique to
  true AP

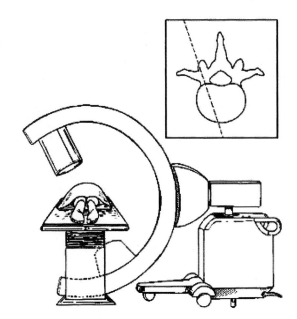

FIGURE 8–9 The direction of the C-arm for the pedicular *en face* view.

needle into the vertebral body relatively safely. Limitations in using the transpedicular approach include inadequate pedicle width, usually above T9, and lateral angulation of the pedicle with respect to the vertebral body. Jamshidi needles (11-gauge) have a 2.5-mm outer diameter. Additionally, vertebral body fractures that are compressed to a level below the pedicles may not be treatable with this approach at this time. In fact, if there is vertebral body compression below the level of pedicles in the thoracic spine, it is difficult to treat it by any procedure or any approach including the extrapedicular approach described below. The reason for this is the high risk of bilateral segmental artery injury. In addition, the transpedicular approach in this

fracture configuration does not allow the instruments to be passed beyond the posterior half of the vertebral body.

The procedure is begun with a small stab wound positioned slightly lateral (~1 cm) to the appropriate pedicle. The spinal needle is directed to the posterior, lateral, superior corner of the pedicle, or centered directly over the pedicle. The former provides the most flexibility in directing the needle.

A 10-degree *en face* fluoroscopy (C-arm) view looking straight down the pedicle (Fig. **8–9**) has the advantage that the physician can visualize the edges of the pedicle and determine that the tool is contained within the pedicle (Fig. **8–10**). With experience, however, some physicians

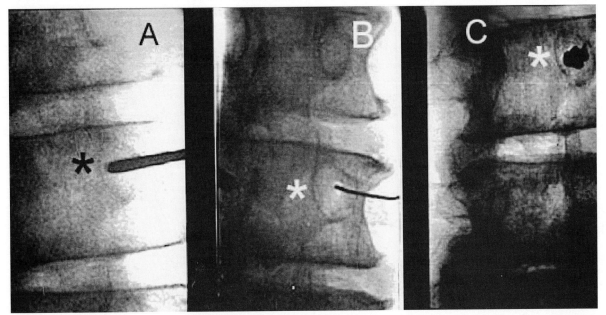

FIGURE 8–10 Tools being introduced into the pedicle using the pedicular *en face* view. **(A)** The 11-gauge needle in the pedicle. **(B)** The guide pin in the pedicle. **(C)** The cannula inside the pedicle.

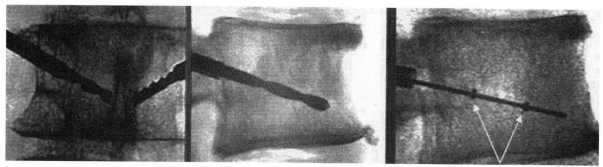

FIGURE 8–11 Tools placed in the inferior half of the vertebral body for superior end-plate fracture. Left anteroposterior x-ray demonstrates drill bits in the final position stopping short of the spinous process and in the inferior half of the vertebral body. Middle lateral x-ray shows final position of the drill bit 3 mm from the anterior cortex and in the inferior half of the vertebral body. Right lateral x-ray shows final placement of the Kyphon inflatable bone tamp. The tamp lies between the two radiographic markers.

use just a true AP view for needle placement to decrease C-arm movement during needle placement in the early parts of the procedure. Prior to advancing the needle anteriorly into the pedicle, the lateral view should be checked to be sure the needle is directed toward the vertebral body. If the patient has a superior fracture, then the tools should be placed inferior to the midline (Fig. **8–11**). If the fracture is through the inferior plate, then the needle should be placed just superior to the midline. If the height of the vertebral body is 1.5 cm or less, the needle should be aimed at the midpoint of the anterior cortex on lateral view. If the height of the vertebral body is less than 9 mm, then the fracture is probably not treatable with the kyphoplasty balloon.

Extrapedicular Approach: Kyphoplasty

In thoracic vertebral bodies from T9 and above, pedicles are narrow and laterally directed. In these vertebra a transpedicular approach results in suboptimal balloon placement, against the lateral cortex instead of near the center of a vertebral body. At these levels an extrapedicular approach is required. The entry point is immediately superior and lateral to the pedicle, just medial to the rib head (or, on occasion, through the rib head) (Fig. **8–12**). With this approach, the pedicle is entered as it connects to the vertebral body slightly laterally. The tools can then be directed to a point just lateral to the center of the vertebral body. If the approach is too lateral, the pulmonary cavity may be entered. If it is too inferior, the segmental artery can be violated.

Posterolateral Approach: Kyphoplasty

In lumbar vertebral bodies with narrow pedicles, or for ease and rapidity of insertion, the posterolateral approach may be used. This is identical to the one described by Ottolenghi[14] for lumbar vertebral biopsies. The skin entry point is 8 to 10 cm lateral to the midline, with the needle directed 40 to 50 degrees from the vertical. The entry point in the bone is at the junction of the pedicle and posterior vertebral body on the lateral fluoroscopic view. Occasionally, this requires a trajectory through the transverse process. This is a safe zone because the exiting nerves are out of harm's way.

A posterolateral approach allows the placement of only one balloon. Less height is achieved with a single balloon. Some loss of height may occur when the balloon is deflated (Fig. **8–13**).

Technical Details: Kyphoplasty

An 11-gauge Jamshidi needle is a convenient way to begin a kyphoplasty, following strategically placed 0.5-cm incisions and the careful insertion technique with multiple fluoroscopic images described above. Once the needle is just inside the posterior cortex of the vertebral body, remove the stylet and insert the guide pin down

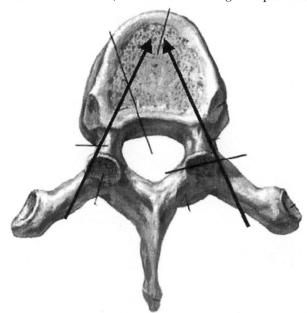

FIGURE 8–12 The extrapedicular entry point.

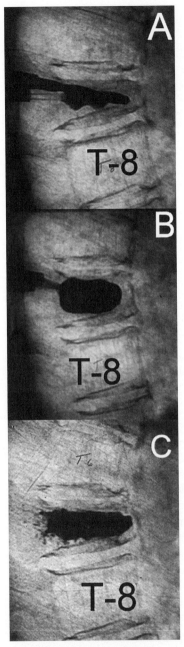

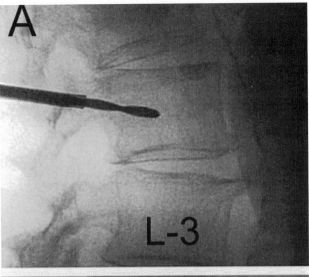

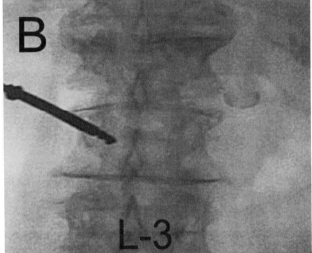

FIGURE 8–14 Anteroposterior (AP) and lateral C-arm images of correct early placement of the drill bit. **(A)** The lateral image with the drill bit halfway across the vertebral body. **(B)** The correct concomitant AP view with the drill bit halfway between the medial edge of the pedicle and the edge of the spinous process.

FIGURE 8–13 (A) Lateral C-arm image of preoperative vertebral body height as balloon begins inflation. **(B)** Vertebral body height is doubled as two balloons are inflated. **(C)** Both balloons were deflated prior to cementation and height improvement was lost.

the shaft of the needle until 1 to 2 mm of the guide pin tip shows. Check placement using a lateral view. Holding the guide pin in place carefully remove the needle and reconfirm guide pin placement with a lateral fluoroscopic view. Advance the blunt dissector over the guide pin. If this requires some force, put the T-handle onto the blunt dissector and tap with a mallet. Do this cautiously to avoid splitting the pedicle, and confirm placement with lateral images. Stop advancing when

the tip of the guide pin is a few millimeters into the vertebral body. Remove the guide pin. Place the cannula over the blunt dissector and advance it just beyond the junction of the pedicle and body on the lateral view using hand pressure or gentle mallet tapping. When the cannula is appropriately placed, remove the blunt dissector and place a drill bit down the cannula. Using manual control, twist the drill bit to enter the vertebral body. The final position is just posterior to the anterior cortex.

When the drill is halfway across the vertebral body in the lateral view, check the AP view to make sure the drill bit is about halfway between the pedicle and the spinous process (Fig. **8–14**). If the drill is too medial on the AP, the spinal canal may be threatened. On the AP view if it

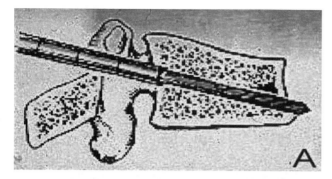

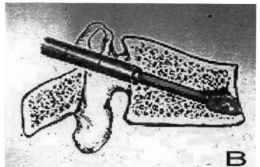

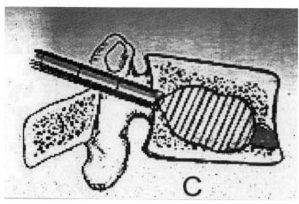

FIGURE 8–15 The procedure for correcting the drill hole in the anterior cortical wall of the vertebral body. If a drill bit is passed too far through the vertebral body **(A)**, then bony putty is passed down into the defect using the bone filler device (BFD) **(B)**. This is done prior to balloon inflation and cementation **(C)**.

is directed straight ahead without any medial deviation, it may advance laterally out of the cortex. On the lateral view it should be within the superior and inferior edge of the pedicle. When the drill bit is positioned appropriately on the image, remove it and insert, through the same cannula, the inflatable bone tamp (IBT).

It should be noted that if the drill bit broaches the anterior cortex of the vertebral body, this must be addressed prior to cementation. The easiest way to plug an anterior cortical hole is to remove the drill bit and pass any bone substitute paste down the cannula with the bone filler device to the defect. Usually 2 or 3 cc are needed to fill the drill hole (Fig. **8–15**).

Inflate the bone tamp with contrast medium (dilution of 60% contrast mixed with saline) using a manometer with a digital pressure gauge to 1 cc or 150 psi, whichever comes first. The initial injection holds the balloon in place while the tools are placed in the contralateral pedicle and another balloon inserted. There should be a gradual reduction of pressure after the bone expands and the cavity is created. Alternate balloon filling should continue until appropriate pressures are reached, and fracture reduction is maximized safely. (See Fig. **8–7** for the inflation sequence and AP and lateral views.) As balloon volumes increase beyond 2 cc, only 0.5 cc or less should be introduced into each balloon until a stopping point is reached.

Fracture reduction using the IBT is guided by (1) desired reduction; (2) proximity of IBT to cortical walls as seen on AP, lateral, and oblique views; (3) pressure read-ings remaining at the maximum of 220 psi (however, see next paragraph); or (4) when maximum rated volumes read from the inflation syringe barrel are reached (4 cc for the 15-mm length or 6 cc for the 20-mm length). With any of these, inflation should stop. Inflate in small-volume increments, alternating sides. Ensure that the IBTs remain inflated with a similar volume, and check for the inflation path and proximity to cortices using frequent AP and lateral views.

There is one further note regarding the maximum pressure of 220 psi. If a balloon is well positioned and no progress has been achieved with a balloon pressure of 220, the surgeon may choose to pressurize beyond this level with careful monitoring. In general, well-controlled and visualized inflations to higher levels, as high as 300 psi, are well tolerated by the balloon. But this technique is only used when cavity formation will be incomplete with the lower pressures.

The risks related to balloon failure are generally minimal. The pressure rapidly decays to zero, a small volume of contrast medium and saline leaks out, and the IBT can be safely removed. On occasion, a torn balloon may be difficult to remove from the vertebral body. Do not pull it out forcibly or the end will break off. Twist the balloon shaft and ease the balloon out. The entire cannula may have to be removed at the same time to successfully remove the balloon.

In addition, contrast medium sensitivity is a precaution but is exceedingly rare. The risks to IBT inflation

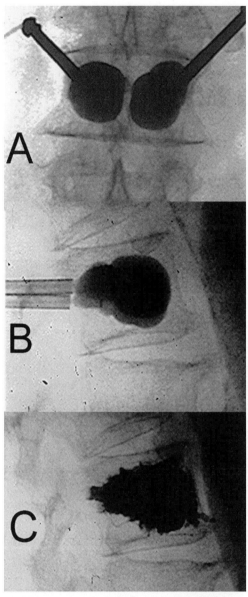

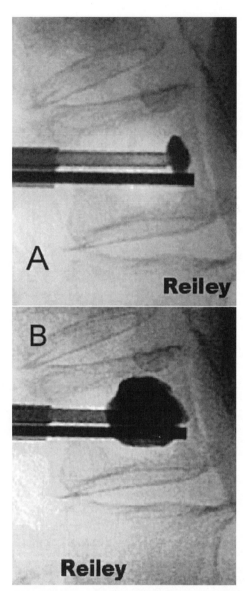

FIGURE 8–16 Cement fill volume is typically greater than the volumes of the inflatable bone tamp (IBT) inflations. Antero-posterior **(A)** and lateral **(B)** views of two IBTs filled to 6 cc each in L2. The eventually cement volume in L2 equaled 14 cc **(C)**. Anterior cement is in an inferior spur.

FIGURE 8–17 Two intraoperative lateral images showing the consistency of cement as it is being injected into the vertebral body cavity: **(A)** 0.5 cc injected; **(B)** 3 cc injected. Note the cement forms a ball because it is so thick at the time of injection.

beyond the cortices are the same as those with a conventional bone tamp and can be avoided by proper placement and careful monitoring.

Once appropriate volume and reduction have occurred, deflate the IBT and slowly rotate and pull out the inflation device. If height elevation of the vertebral body has occurred, then the surgeon may keep one balloon elevated while the other balloon is removed. Usually the balloon with the highest pressure is left inflated. Further, that balloon should remain elevated while the opposite cavity is filled with the bone filler. If cement is used, once the cement is extremely doughy and thick, it should be able to support the vertebral body height and the

other balloon can be deflated and removed and the cavity filled.

There are currently no commercially available bone cement mixtures with enough barium to allow visualization during cement injection. Therefore, additional sterile barium must be added to the mixture. To accomplish this, it is recommended that 6 g of sterile barium be mixed with polymethylmethacrylate (PMMA) powder before adding the liquid monomer. Normally, within a minute, the mix goes from powdery to a thick, soupy consistency.

If PMMA is chosen by the treating physician, powder measured to 40 cc in a 60-cc syringe should be mixed with 6 g of sterile barium (Bryan Corp., Woburn, MA) in a mixing bowl. Add 5 cc of liquid monomer for every 20 cc of powder, mix with a spatula for 1 minute, and pour into four or five 5-cc syringes with the plungers removed. Remove the stylet from the Kyphon cement cannula (bone filler device, BFD) and attach the nozzle to the Luer of the 5-cc syringes. Each cement cannula holds 1.5 cc. Knowing the volume of the void from the volume of the IBT inflations, fill enough BFDs to exceed that volume by 1 to 8 cc depending on the size of the vertebral body, the interdigitation of the cement, and the constant vigilance of the surgeon on multiple C-arm views (Fig. **8–16**).

The lumbar spine vertebral bodies may accept more cement than is needed for thoracic vertebrae. Thoracic vertebral bodies require ~40 cc of powder; lumbar bodies require 60 cc of powder. If there is any doubt about the size of the vertebral body, mix more, rather than less, cement. It can be frustrating to have an excellent balloon reduction and cavity formation only to have an insufficient amount of cement to fill the vertebral body. It is not usual to fill a lumbar vertebral body with 12 to 16 cc of cement.

Whatever filler is chosen, the appropriate viscosity needs to be achieved prior to application. Fillers should have the consistency of caulking material. For example, the consistency of PMMA should be stiff, without sheen, and no dripping from the end of the mixing spatula (Fig. **8–17**). This viscosity may occur in 7 to 15 minutes, depending on the cement additives and room temperature. The ability to place materials with high viscosity significantly reduces the risk of leaks (Fig. **8–18**).

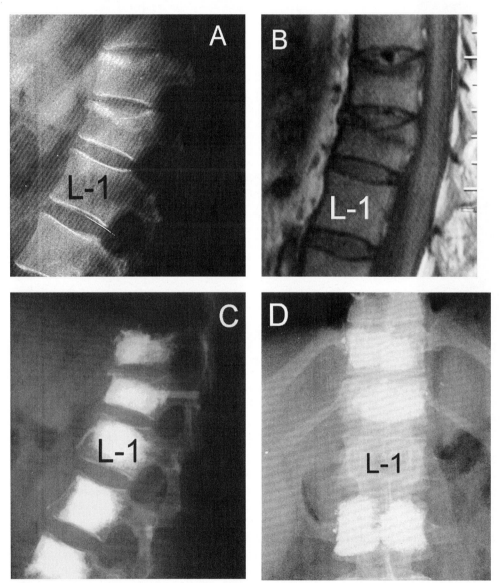

FIGURE 8–18 Four views of pre- and postcementation in a 34-year-old woman with severe osteoporosis due to 20 years of bulimia. Patient seized and fractured six vertebral bodies. Lateral views of the fractures on plain x-ray **(A)** and magnetic resonance imaging **(B)**, **(C)** and anteroposterior **(D)** views postcementation are shown. T11 and T12 were filled with 10 and 12 cc, respectively, and L1 and L2 were filled with 14 and 16 cc, respectively. Cement was extremely firm at the time of injection to prevent leakage.

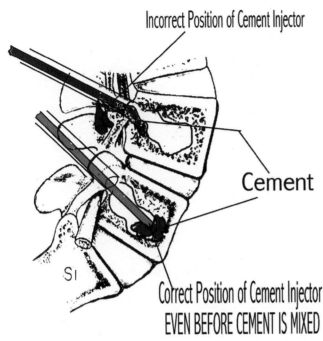

Incorrect Position of Cement Injector

Cement

Correct Position of Cement Injector
EVEN BEFORE CEMENT IS MIXED

FIGURE 8–19 Proper placement of the cement cannula. The cannula must be entered all the way into the anterior portion of the cavity to begin cementation. If left inside the pedicle, cement will leak into the canal.

When ready to fill, one (if some height restoration is achieved) or both IBTs are deflated and, using lateral C-arm guidance, a cement cannula (BFD) is inserted through the working cannula to the anterior wall of the vertebral body. Confirm placement on AP and lateral images. Improper placement of the cement cannula can lead to leakage into the spinal canal (Fig. **8–19**). The cement cannula stylet is used to gently push the selected viscous bone filler from the cement cannula while the cement cannula is withdrawn to the level of the middle of the cavity. With continued low-pressure injection, the volume of the cement grows around the BFD as it is held in place in the middle of the void. Leaks generally do not occur unless the bone filler is too runny or a cortex was violated. If filler begins to escape anteriorly or through the end plates, stop injecting for 90 seconds or so. Repeat the process from side to side if necessary.

The greatest risk is associated with posterior leakage. At the first sign of cement entering the pedicles or approaching 2 to 3 mm of the posterior vertebral body cortex, injection should be stopped. If the cement is still runny, or even slightly runny, no further injection should be performed until the cement has set up further. Once the cement has become much less viscous it may be safe to inject further cement with the cement cannula advanced well anteriorly in the vertebral body. If the surgeon can visualize cement interdigitating into the superior, inferior, or anterior portion of the vertebral body, and no cement advancing posteriorly, further cement injection can slowly be performed.

The cannulas should be twisted and removed prior to the cement becoming hard. If cement has set up a little, it is still possible to remove the cannula by slightly flexing it to break off any filler in its distal tip and then pulling out. Obtain final AP and lateral x-rays to ensure that no filler has gone into the canal. Leave the patient in position on the table until the cement has hardened; usually when the cement outside the body in the mixing cup is hard, then the cement is sufficiently polymerized to allow the patient to be moved off the table. Suture or Steri-Strip the wound.

■ Postoperative Care

This patient population is typically frail and vulnerable, so many patients are admitted to the hospital for overnight monitoring. Elderly men with compression fractures typically have benign prostatic hypertrophy and need to be monitored for appropriate urine output. They are encouraged to resume all their typical daily activities as soon as feasible with no restrictions, except lifting. Only limited lifting is permitted for 6 weeks. This is to prevent fractures at the untreated levels, which is demoralizing to a patient in the early postoperative period. Patients are examined at 1 week to check the wound, and then at 2 weeks postoperation to determine if truncal strengthening needs to be instituted with a physical therapist. This back-strengthening program is almost always required, especially for gluteus maximus strengthening. At 3-month intervals the patient is reexamined to ensure other fractures are not developing. All patients are started on systemic osteoporosis treatment (vitamin D, calcium, and antiresorptive agents) and encouraged to participate in some form of tolerable exercise program for life.

■ Outcomes and Complications

Vertebroplasty data from about 400 patients have been reported in several case series.[15–20] The longest reported follow-up is 3 years, although the first paper on vertebroplasty was published in 1986. Reportedly, pain has been reduced in 70 to 90% of patients. There have been no reported cement failures, and only two reported cases of fracture progression in the treated vertebral bodies (caused by inadequate cement fill). Cement leakage rates have been reported to occur in 34 to 67% of cases,[13,21–25] but is usually clinically insignificant. Reported major complications due to cement leaks include increased pain, radiculopathies, pulmonary embolism, and spinal cord compression. Cement leakage leading to radiculopathy or spinal cord injury is more common following the treatment of pathologic fractures resulting from metastasis than for osteoporotic fractures.

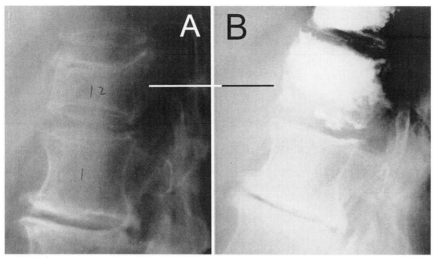

FIGURE 8–20 T11 and T12 fractures in a 260-pound 70-year-old woman. Fractures were treated at 33 days postinjury. **(A)** Lateral preoperative x-ray of T12 fractured down to 1.5 cm. **(B)** Postoperative lateral x-ray with the T12 height improved to 4 cm. Note small amount of leakage in the inferior disk.

The most recent vertebroplasty report from the United State involves 47 patients with an average follow-up of 18 months.[26] The report outlines marked to complete pain relief in only 63% of patients with osteoporotic vertebral compression fractures. Their results with osteolytic metastatic vertebral collapse in eight patients revealed that only four patients experienced any pain relief. In this group of patients there was a 6% complication rate.

The first kyphoplasty was performed in September 1998, and by April 2001 over 3000 patients in the United States have had kyphoplasty procedures. Well over 90% of patients reported significant pain relief. In prospective multicenter series there were six major complications (1.1%), four of which were neurologic complications

(0.75%). These were directly attributable to surgeon error and breach of technique.

In a phase one institutional review board approved study just recently completed at the Cleveland Clinic, 64 consecutive kyphoplasty procedures were performed in 29 patients over 34 sessions.[27] The mean age was 68.6 years (range 48–86). The indications included painful primary ($n = 19$) or secondary ($n = 4$) osteoporotic vertebral compression fractures in a total of 20 patients unresponsive to nonoperative modalities. A further five patients presented with painful compression fractures due to multiple myeloma. The mean duration of symptoms was 3.5 months (range 0.5–12). Outcome data were obtained by comparing preoperative and latest

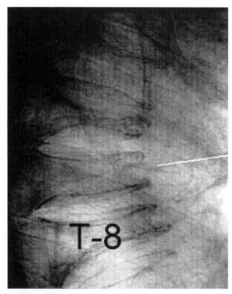
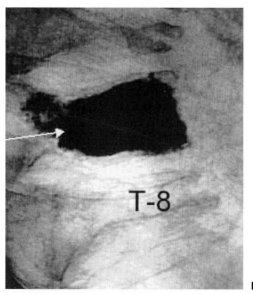

A   B

FIGURE 8–21 Multiple thoracic fractures in an 82-year-old woman. **(A)** Prekyphoplasty lateral x-ray shows T7 to be 1 cm in height. T6 and T8 are less than 9 mm and are not treatable by kyphoplasty. **(B)** Excellent correction of height to 2.3 cm. (Courtesy of Eeric Truumees, MD, William Beaumont Hospital, Michigan.)

postoperative Health Status Questionnaire Short-Form 36 (SF-36) data. In this study all 25 patients tolerated the procedure well, and improvement in pain and mobility was seen early. Virtually all patients subjectively reported immediate relief of their typical fracture pain, and no patient complained of worse pain at the treated levels. The levels treated ranged from T6 to L5, the majority at the thoracolumbar junction (T11, $n = 7$; T12, $n = 14$; L1, $n = 9$). Seventy percent of the levels treated showed a 47% restoration of the lost height. Thirty percent of the levels treated showed no appreciable height restoration even though generous cavities were created within the collapsed vertebral bodies. SF-36 scores for the Bodily Pain, Physical Function, Vitality, and Role Physical subscales all showed statistically significant improvement. At final follow-up there were five clinically insignificant cement leaks (8% overall), and no major systemic complications or neurologic injuries related directly to use of this technique or the inflatable bone tamp.

In general, height restitution, as mentioned above, is difficult to predict preoperatively, and the patient should be warned of that. Early fractures are extremely well treated, and height improvement is quite rewarding to the surgeon and the patient (Figs. 8–20 and 8–21).

Kyphoplasty by creating a cavity and realigning the spine appears to have significant advantages over vertebroplasty. Kyphoplasty minimizes the risk of cement leakage by compacting the cancellous bone to the periphery and sealing off the fracture clefts, and by creating a cavity into which cement is packed as opposed to injected under pressure. This technique may prevent propagation of further fractures by reducing the collapsed vertebral bodies toward their native height and thus normalizing the sagittal spinal alignment. Both techniques have proven to be a valuable tool in the treatment of painful progressive osteoporotic compression fractures.

REFERENCES

1. Cooper C, Atkinson EJ, O'Fallon WM, Melton LJ III. Incidence of clinically diagnosed vertebral fractures: a population-based study in Rochester, Minnesota, 1985–1989. J Bone Miner Res 1992;7:221–227
2. Riggs,BL, Melton,LJ III. The worldwide problem of osteoporosis: insights afforded by epidemiology. BONE 1995;17(5 Suppl):505S-511S
3. Leech JA, Dulberg C, Kellie S, Pattee L, Gay J. Relationship of lung function to severity of osteoporosis in women. Am Rev Respir Dis 1990;141:68–71
4. Silverman S. The clinical consequences of vertebral compression fracture. Bone 1992;13:S27–S32
5. Cook DJ, Guyatt GH, Adachi JD, et al, and the Multicentre Vertebral Fracture Study Group. Quality of life issues in women with vertebral fractures due to osteoporosis. Arthritis Rheum 1993;36:750–756
6. Lyles, KW, Gold DT, Shipp KM, et al. Association of osteoporotic vertebral fractures with impaired functional status. Am J Med 1993;94:595–598
7. Schlaich C, Minne HW, Bruckner T, et al. Reduced pulmonary function in patients with spinal osteoporotic fractures. Osteoporos Int 1998;8:261–267
8. Nevitt MC, Ettinger B, Black DM, et al. The association of radiographically detected vertebral fractures with back pain and function: a prospective study. Ann Intern Med 1998;128:793–800
9. Oleksik A, Lips P, Dawson A, et al. Health-related quality of life in postmenopausal women with low BMD with or without prevalent vertebral fractures. J Bone Miner Res 2000;15:1384–1392
10. Kado DM, Browner WS, Palermo L, Nevitt MC, Genant HK, Cummings SR. Vertebral fractures and mortality in older women: a prospective study. Study of Osteoporotic Fractures Research Group. Arch Intern Med 1999;159:1215–1220
11. Cooper C, Atkinson EJ, Jacobsen SJ, et al. Incidence of clinically diagnosed vertebral fractures: a population-based study in Rochester, Minnesota, 1985–1989. J Bone Miner Res 1993;7:221–227
12. Galibert P, Deramond H, Rosat P, Le Gars D. [Preliminary note on the treatment of vertebral angioma by percutaneous acrylic vertebroplasty] (in French). Neurochirurgie 1987;33:166–168.
13. Jensen ME, Evans AJ, Mathis JM, Kallmes DF, Cloft HJ, Dion JE. Percutaneous polymethylmethacrylate verterboplasty in the treatment of osteoporotic vertebral body compression fractures: technical aspects. AJNR Am J Neuroradiol 1997;18:1897–1904
14. Ottolenghi CE. Aspiration biopsy of the spine: technique for the thoracic spine and results of twenty-eight biopsies in this region and over-all results of 1050 biopsies of other spinal segments. J Bone Joint Surg Am 1969;51:1531–1544
15. Cotton, C, Dewatre F, Cortet, B, et al. Percutaneous vertebroplasty for osteolytic metastasis and myeloma: effects of the percentage of lesion filling and the leakage of methylmetacrylate at clinical follow-up. RADIOL 1996;200:525–530
16. Cortet B, Cotton A, Boutry N, et al. Percutaneous vertebroplasty in patients with Osteolytic metastases or multiple myeloma. Rev Rhum 1997;64:177–183
17. Weill A, Chirs J, Simon JM, et al. Spinal metastases: indications for and results of percutaneous injection of surgical cement. Radiol 1996;199:241–247
18. Jensen ME, Evans AJ, Mathis, et al. Percutaneous polymethylmethacrylate verterboplasty in the treatment of osteoporotic vertebral body compression fractures: technical aspects. Am J Neuroradiol 1997;18:1897–1904
19. Martin J B, Jean B, Sugiu K, et al. Vertebroplasty: clinical experience and follow-up results. Bone 1999;25:11S-15S.
20. Deramond H, Depriester C, Galibert P, Le Gars D. Percutaneous vertebroplasty with polymethylmethacrylate: technique, indications and results. Radiol Clin North Am 1998;36:533–546
21. Cotton A, Dewatre F, Cortet B, et al. Percutaneous vertebroplasty for osteolytic metastases and myeloma: effects of the percentage of lesion filling and the leakage of methyl methacrylate at clinical follow-up. Radiology 1996;200:525–530
22. Weill A, Chiras J, Simon JM, Rose M, Sola-Martinez T, Enkaoua E. Spinal metastases: indications for and results of percutaneous injection of acrylic surgical cement. Radiology 1996;199:241–247
23. Padovani B, Kasriel O, Brunner P, et al. Pulmonary embolism caused acrylic cement: a rare complication of percutaneous vertebroplasty. Am J Neuroradiol 1999;20:375–377
24. Deramond H, Depriester C, Galibert P, et al. Percutaneous vertebroplasty with polymethymethacrylate: technique, indications and results. Radiol Clin N Am 1998;36:533–546
25. Chiras J, Depriester C, Weill A, Sola-Martinez MT, Deramond H. [Percutaneous vertebral surgery: techniques and indications] (in French). J Neuroradiol 1997;24:45–59
26. Barr JD, Barr MS, Lemley TJ, et al. Spine 2000;25:923–928
27. Lieberman IH, Dudeney S, Reinhardt MK, Bell GR. Initial outcome and efficacy of kyphoplasty in the treatment of painful osteoporotic vertebral compression fractures. Spine 2001;26:1631–1638.
28. Padovani B, Kasriel O, Brunner P, Peretti-Viton P. Pulmonary embolism caused by acrylic cement: a rare complication of percutaneous vertebroplasty. AJNR Am J Neuroradiol 1999;20:375–377

9

Clinical Results of Kyphoplasty in the Treatment of Osteoporotic and Osteolytic Vertebral Compression Fractures

ISADOR LIEBERMAN

Objectives: On completion of this chapter, the reader should be able to discuss the differences between kyphoplasty and vertebroplasty.

Accreditation: The American Association of Neurological Surgeons is accredited by the Accreditation Council for Continuing Medical Education to sponsor continuing medical education for physicians.

Credit: The American Association of Neurological Surgeons designates this continuing medical education activity for a maximum of 15 credits in Category I of the Physician's Recognition Award of the American Medical Association.

The Home Study Examination is online at www.aans.org/education/books/vertebro.asp

Kyphoplasty is a new technique in the treatment of osteoporotic or osteolytic painful progressive vertebral wedge compression fractures (VCFs). This technique, conceived and developed by Mark Reiley, M.D. (Berkley, California), has several benefits and potential advantages over historical and current treatment modalities for VCFs. It involves the introduction of a cannula into the vertebral body, followed by insertion of an inflatable bone tamp (IBT) designed to elevate the end plates and reduce the vertebral body back toward its original height, while creating a cavity to be filled with bone cement. By reducing the vertebral body back toward its native height, the sagittal alignment of the spine is restored, providing patients with cosmetic and functional improvement, as well as potentially protecting other levels from collapse due to the force transmission associated with a kyphotic posture. By creating a cavity, the cement augmentation is performed with more control into the low-pressure environment of the preformed cavity with viscous, partially cured cement, thereby reducing the risk of cement extravasation. By stabilizing the vertebral body, pain from the progressive fracture collapse or the altered biomechanics can be minimized or even eliminated. From its introduction in 1998 to June 2001, over 3000 patients have been treated at several

centers in the United States. Due to limited (timewise) experience, however, only a few reports have been presented at national and international meetings and only one peer-reviewed and two invited publications appear in the literature. The early data from these reports indicate that kyphoplasty has a significant positive effect on pain relief, deformity, and quality of life.

■ Outcomes

As with any medical intervention, clinical outcome is inextricably linked to patient selection based on strict indications. The indications for kyphoplasty are painful or progressive osteoporotic and osteolytic vertebral compression fractures. The contraindications include systemic pathologies such as sepsis, prolonged bleeding times, and cardiopulmonary pathology, which would preclude the safe completion of the procedure under either conscious sedation or general anesthesia. Other relative contraindications include nonosteolytic infiltrative spinal metastases, vertebral bodies with deficient posterior cortices, and neurologic symptoms or signs. In certain burst, or vertebra plana, fracture configurations, kyphoplasty may be technically difficult, and the feasibility of the procedure should be assessed on the merits of the individual case.

Kyphoplasty procedures have been performed by over 400 surgeons for over 5000 vertebral compression fractures. From information gathered by Kyphon Inc. in a prospective fashion, and reported by Garfin et al[1] over 90% of the patients reported significant pain relief after kyphoplasty. The procedures were performed under either local or general anesthesia and were well tolerated. In the first 600 patients, there were six major complications (1%), four of which were neurologic complications (0.75%). These were directly attributable to surgeon error and breach of technique. None of these complications were attributable to the IBT.

In an introductory article Wong et al[2] reported that 80 of 85 patients (94%) treated with kyphoplasty experienced good to excellent pain relief as measured with a pain questionnaire. In this series one patient had a presumed cement embolus to the lungs. This occurred early in the kyphoplasty experience, when highly runny cement was used. They go on to report that the cementing technique has been modified and tools have been developed to allow for placement of viscous, partially cured cement into the vertebral body. They also report that after kyphoplasty anterior vertebral body height increased from 79% ± 22% to 99% ± 13% of estimated normal anterior height.

Phillips and McNally[3] reported excellent pain relief in a series of 40 patients treated with kyphoplasty. They did not encounter any major systemic complications or neurologic injuries. In those patients in whom they were able to achieve fracture reduction, they noted that the local segmental kyphosis was improved by a mean of 14 degrees.

In their initial phase one institutional review board approved study, Lieberman et al[4] reported on 70 consecutive kyphoplasty procedures performed in 30 patients over 38 operative sessions. The indications in this group included painful primary ($n = 19$), or secondary ($n = 5$), osteoporotic vertebral compression fractures for a total of 24 patients unresponsive to nonoperative modalities. A further six patients presented with painful compression fractures due to multiple myeloma. The duration of symptoms ranged from 0.5 to 24 months (average 5.9 months). Symptomatic levels were identified by correlating the physical findings with radiographic evidence of collapse and with magnetic resonance imaging (MRI) findings of marrow signal changes consistent with compression fractures. Outcome data were prospectively collected by comparing preoperative and latest postoperative Health Status Questionnaire Short-Form 36 (SF-36) data. Height restoration was assessed by comparing a single midline vertebral body height measurement on pre- and postoperative radiographs.

In this study all 30 patients tolerated the procedure well, and improvement in pain and mobility was seen early. Virtually all patients subjectively reported immediate relief of their typical fracture pain and no patient complained of worse pain at the treated levels. The levels treated ranged from T6 to L5, with the majority at the thoracolumbar junction. Height measurement from plain radiographs of all 70 levels treated (regardless of fracture age) demonstrated that in 70% of the vertebral bodies, kyphoplasty restored 47% of the lost height. Thirty percent of the levels treated showed no appreciable height restoration, even though generous cavities were created within the collapsed vertebral bodies. Cement extravasation was noted in only six vertebral bodies (9%) in the early cases. None resulted in any clinical consequences. The SF-36 scores for the Bodily Pain, Physical Function, Role Physical, Vitality, and Mental Health subscales all showed statistically significant improvement, either reaching or approaching the age-matched SF-36 historical controls. At final follow-up there were no major complications related directly to the use of this technique or the inflatable bone tamp.

In a continued prospective follow-up of the first 60 patients out to a minimum of 24 weeks, the SF-36 scores maintained their statistically significant improvement in every category, except general health and role emotional, which maintained their level at the age-matched norm (Fig. 9–1).

Dudeney et al[5] presented their initial experience in 18 patients using the kyphoplasty technique to treat osteolytic compression fractures secondary to multiple myeloma. The indications for treatment were painful progressive osteolytic compression fractures. In this group all patients had multiple level involvement, and on average had five levels treated over three surgical sessions. The levels treated ranged from T7 to L5, the majority at the thoracolumbar junction. All patients tolerated the procedure well. Improvement in pain and mobility was seen early. Most patients reported immediate relief of their typical fracture pain. None complained of worse pain at the treated levels. No problems were encountered in those patients undergoing concurrent chemotherapy or radiotherapy. The mean central vertebral height lost was 8.4 mm (range 2–18 mm). The mean percentage of height lost that was restored by the procedure was 30% (range 0–73%). The authors felt that the difference in height restoration compared with their cohort of osteoporotic patients was due to the difference in fracture configuration. Whereas the majority of osteoporotic fractures are true wedge compression fractures, the myeloma fractures are typically biconcave end-plate deformities. The osteolytic fractures also tend to progress over a longer time frame and thus may actually be subject to some remodeling depending on how well the myeloma is controlled. In this group cement extravasation was seen at two levels (8.6%). SF-36 scores after a minimum follow-up of 6 months for the subscales Bodily

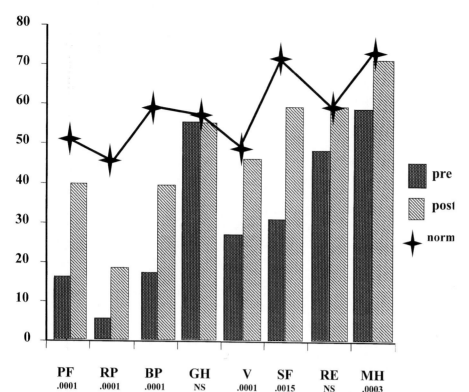

PF RP BP GH V SF RE MH
.0001 .0001 .0001 NS .0001 .0015 NS .0003

Figure 9–1 Results of kyphoplasty and SF-36 questionnaire outcome, $n = 60$, follow-up at 24 weeks.

Pain (14.2 to 56.8, $p = .0091$), Physical Function (11.2 to 56.2, $p = .014$), Role Physical (0 to 28.1, $p = .47$), Vitality (23.8 to 45.6, $p = .042$), and Social Functioning (30.6 to 68.1, $p = .015$) all showed improvement. At final follow-up there were no major complications in the myeloma patients related directly to use of this technique or the inflatable bone tamp.

■ Conclusion

These initial results show that kyphoplasty is a well-tolerated procedure indicated for the treatment of painful progressive osteoporotic or osteolytic vertebral compression fractures. Kyphoplasty is associated with a statistically significant improvement in pain and function, as well as restoration of vertebral body height, with a low risk of cement extravasation. It appears that like hip fracture surgery, kyphoplasty will be most successful with early intervention.

REFERENCES

1. Garfin SR, Yuan H, Lieberman IH, et al. Early results of 300 kyphoplasties for the treatment of painful vertebral body compression fractures. Proceedings AAOS annual meeting, San Francisco, March 2001
2. Wong W, Reiley MA, Garfin S. Vertebroplasty/kyphoplasty. J Women's Imaging 2000;2:117–124
3. Phillips FM, McNally T. Early clinical and radiographic results for kyphoplasty in the treatment of osteopenic vertebral compression fractures. Proceedings ISSLS annual meeting, Edinburgh, June 2001
4. Lieberman I, Dudeney S, Reinhardt MK, Bell G. Initial outcome and efficacy of kyphoplasty in the treatment of painful osteoporotic vertebral compression fractures. Spine 2001;26:1631–1638
5. Dudeney S, Hussein MA, Karam MA, Reinhardt MK, Lieberman IH. "Kyphoplasty" in the treatment of Osteolytic Vertebral Fractures secondary to Multiple Myeloma. Proceedings NASS annual meeting, Seattle, November 2001.

10

Complication Avoidance and Management in Vertebroplasty and Kyphoplasty

H. CLAUDE SAGI, GEOFFREY MCCULLEN, AND HANSEN A. YUAN

Objectives: On completion of this chapter, the reader should be able to describe the results reported in the literature regarding patients treated with kyphoplasty.

Accreditation: The American Association of Neurological Surgeons is accredited by the Accreditation Council for Continuing Medical Education to sponsor continuing medical education for physicians.

Credit: The American Association of Neurological Surgeons designates this continuing medical education activity for a maximum of 15 credits in Category I of the Physician's Recognition Award of the American Medical Association.

The Home Study Examination is online at www.aans.org/education/books/vertebro.asp

---

Although the steps of both vertebroplasty and kyphoplasty are simple in concept, the technical demands are great. The technical aspects of each technique are discussed elsewhere in this book. However, the essential difference between the two techniques (high-pressure injection of low-viscosity cement versus low-pressure injection of high-viscosity cement, respectively) underscores the theoretical risks of complications. Complication avoidance requires strict adherence to guidelines for patient selection, instrument placement, and filling technique. When performed in the operating room, the anesthesia team needs to be informed of the unique issues pertinent to these procedures.

■ Vertebroplasty: Reported and Potential Complications

The majority of the complications from vertebroplasty procedures result from cement extravasation out of the confines of the vertebral body (cement leaks). High pressures are used to deliver polymethylmethacrylate (PMMA) in a relatively low viscosity because it must displace the intratrabecular contents. Cement leaks are relatively common (up to 67%),[1] but reported complications are few. Possible scenarios include foraminal and soft

tissue leaks associated with increased pain[1] and/or radiculopathy,[1–4] venous leaks associated with pulmonary embolism with infarction,[5] and intradiskal leaks that have not been reported to lead to complications. Epidural leaks into the spinal canal are the most devastating because they can lead to spinal cord injury.[6,7] This can occur secondary to misplaced instruments (Fig. 10–1), or leakage through discontinuities in the posterior wall (Fig. 10–2). The reported rate of neurologic injury for the treatment of osteoporotic fractures with vertebroplasty is 1.3% for radiculopathy and <0.5% for cord compression.[6]

Moreland et al[8] reported on the complications and techniques to avoid them in their first 50 patients. Cement extravasation occurred in 8% (four patients), and necessitated posterior open decompression in three because of epidural extension. Two patients had symptomatic pulmonary emboli of methylmethacrylate, and one patient had a cerebrospinal fluid (CSF) leak that was treated with bed rest for a total complication rate of 14%. In Jensen et al's[9] study of 47 fractures in 29 patients, two patients sustained rib fractures, two patients had PMMA extravasation into the vena cava, and one patient had extravasation into the epidural space. There were no adverse sequelae related to these complications. Deramond et al[3] reported only

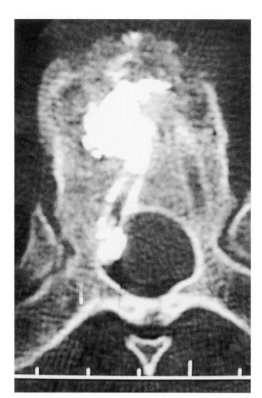

FIGURE 10–1 Axial computed tomography (CT) scan showing cement leak through errant trocar path.

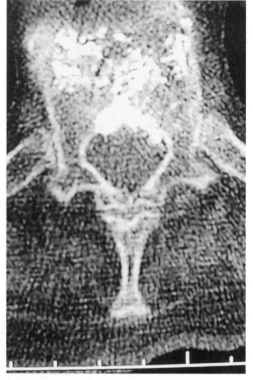

FIGURE 10–2 Axial computed tomography (CT) scan showing cement leak through breach in posterior vertebral body.

one patient in 80 with an intercostal neuralgia. Wenger et al[7] had one patient in 13 who developed a severe neurologic deterioration following posterior leakage of PMMA into the spinal canal. They now recommend open surgical placement of the needle and filling with cement. Cyteval et al[10] had a 5% complication rate. One patient in 20 had extravasation into the psoas muscle with persistent crural pain. Martin et al[11] quote a 6% incidence of complications per level treated, due primarily to leakage, poor patient evaluation, positioning, and anesthesia. Cortet et al[12] found that extravasation was frequent, occurring in 11 of 16 patients (seven paravertebral muscle, three epidural, and one lumbar venous plexus) but no clinically relevant sequelae resulted. Barr et al[13] reported two patients out of 38 with a complication. One patient developed neuritis secondary to foraminal extravasation, and one patient developed an adjacent fracture.

Pulmonary complications related to injection of PMMA are rare. Padovani et al[5] reported a case of a patient with pulmonary embolism of PMMA to the lung causing infarction. The patient was treated successfully with anticoagulation. Apparently perivertebral venous migration had not been recognized at the time of injection due to the use of lateral imaging only. Systemic falls in arterial pressure such as that seen with cementation of femoral

prostheses in hip arthroplasty[14,15] has not been seen with vertebroplasty.

■ Metastatic and Primary Tumors of the Spine

Neurologic complications can occur at higher rates in patients with metastatic disease (up to 10%).[1,6] Deramond et al[20] have treated 88 patients with vertebral angiomata using percutaneous vertebroplasty; there were two complications (2.3%) of postoperative neuralgia.[3] For malignant spinal tumors (primary and secondary), vertebroplasty is indicated when collapse is not more than two thirds of the initial height, there is no epidural involvement or neurologic deficit, and pain persists despite appropriate medical therapy without evidence of instability. The complication rate related to cement leakage does tend to be higher, with a reported 10% in this group of patients.

Weill et al[1] reported on the use of vertebroplasty to treat painful metastatic lesions of the spine. There was a 9% complication rate related to cement extrusion and radiculopathy. Cotton et al[2] reported that cement leak occurred in 73% (38% epidural), but only three cases resulted in radiculopathy. Interestingly, Barr et al[13] found no complications in their group of nine patients with spinal metastases.

Other complications generally relate to patient selection and technical issues. These are postoperative hematoma, infection,[6] rib fractures,[9] and skin lesions or pressure ulceration. Peh et al[16] have also stated that there are unpublished reports of massive hemorrhage requiring transfusion, as well as patient deaths, possibly due to instrument misplacement. This is supported by reports to the Food and Drug Administration (FDA) under the Medical Device Reporting system of four patient deaths during vertebroplasty.[17]

■ Complication Avoidance in Vertebroplasty

Complication avoidance can be grouped into three general categories: patient selection, training, and technique.

Patient Selection

Vertebroplasty is safely performed in the subacute phase 3 to 4 weeks after fracture occurrence.[18] Fracture lines and defects are not yet sealed by hematoma and fracture callus. Blood vessel damage as well as angiogenesis result in fragile vasculature prone to injury. Risk of cement leaks and perioperative bleeding are increased with acute fractures. Any patient with a neurologic deficit attributable to the compression fracture should not have the procedure.

Appropriate preoperative imaging is essential to rule out fractures or defects in the posterior wall of the vertebral body, as well as extrusion of bone or disk material into the canal. Other contraindications include active infection and, in some cases, solid metastatic tumors.

Preoperative blood work should be drawn to exclude coagulopathy. Any coagulopathy should be corrected to an international normalized ratio (INR) of less than 1.2.

Training

Attendance at a course run by expert faculty that includes a thorough, hands on, cadaver experience should be a prerequisite prior to performing this technique. Expertise in spinal surgery and/or image-guided spinal techniques should also be required. Peh et al[16] believe that the serious, anecdotal complications occur with untrained or poorly trained practitioners. This is supported by the Medical Device Reporting to the FDA not reflected in the clinical literature.[17]

Technique

Frequent use of lateral and anteroposterior fluoroscopic images to guide needle placement helps reduce the risk of complications related to misplacement of the needle. Prior to injection of the PMMA, some authors[9,11] advocate venography by injection of radiocontrast to exclude needle placement into the basivertebral plexus and avoid the potential risk of pulmonary or epidural extravasation of PMMA. Placement of the needle within the plexus is indicated by rapid washout of contrast material.

Continuous lateral fluoroscopic images should be used when injecting the PMMA. Adequate radiopacity aids in PMMA visualization. Current PMMA formulations do not contain enough barium; therefore, it is recommended that 6 g of sterile barium (Bryan Corp., Woburn, MA) be added to 40 cc of Cranioplast PMMA powder (Johnson & Johnson Codman, Raynham, MA), and 10 cc Cranioplast monomer. Cranioplast is the PMMA of choice because of its long working life. It must be loaded into numerous 1-cc syringes as soon as it reaches the liquid state, and used quickly before it hardens. The high pressures required to fill the vertebral body and force the low-viscosity PMMA into the interstices of the trabeculae make the risk of leaks very high (reported up to 70%).

To minimize leaks, it is recommended to place the injection needles as anterior as possible, and to stop the fill when the cement is two thirds of the way back to the posterior wall. It is also recommended that, when a leak occurs, to stop immediately, move the syringe back a millimeter, wait for the local cement to harden, and then continue to fill. If there is still a leak, filling on that side should cease. Several cement guns are available for PMMA injection using vertebroplasty. This allows more viscous cement to be used but involves much higher pressures. If there is a leak while using the gun, the nozzle is immediately turned backward to prevent the pressure wave from continuing to push the cement into the vertebral body. Treating no more than three levels at a time in a single patient is a prudent choice to control the patient's exposure to PMMA monomer and decrease the risk of cement leaks. Two of the patient deaths reported in the FDA Medical Device Reporting system occurred in patients who had seven and 11 levels treated in one operation.

Techniques to avoid complications were suggested by Moreland et al's[8] presentation at the North American Spine Society (NASS) conference in New Orleans, October 2000. They recommend preoperative computed tomography (CT) scan to assess pedicle size and posterior wall continuity. In addition, they recommend preinjection venograms, unilateral injection only for the majority, and injection when the cement is in a higher viscosity state.

No patient should be moved until the PMMA has hardened in the container in which it was mixed, and final x-ray views confirm that no cement is in the canal. Patients are kept on flat bed rest for at least 4 hours, at which point the PMMA has hardened to 90% of its maximum strength.

The risk of infection can potentially be reduced with the use of preoperative antibiotic and the addition of antibiotic to the PMMA powder prior to adding the monomer.[9]

In patients with severe osteoporosis, attention to patient positioning may prevent rib fractures. Additionally, care must be taken not to be too forceful or aggressive with needle application because rib fractures have been known to occur. Appropriate padding and positioning help to minimize pressure ulcerations.

■ Kyphoplasty: Reported and Potential Complications

Kyphoplasty involves minimally invasive reduction and stabilization of a vertebral body compression fracture. Reduction is performed with an inflatable bone tamp (balloon). Balloon inflation creates a void and compacts the surrounding bone. The presence of the cavity thus created allows PMMA or another chosen filler to be injected into the void under lower pressure in a relatively high viscosity state. This low-pressure high-viscosity injection potentially reduces the risk of cement leakage and its attendant complications.

In a cadaveric study comparing vertebroplasty and kyphoplasty, Belkoff et al[19] showed that five of eight vertebral bodies leaked in the vertebroplasty group, whereas zero of eight vertebral bodies leaked in the kyphoplasty group. In a clinical series, Lieberman et al[20] reported six leaks in 70 vertebral bodies (8.3%).

To date there have been four reported neurologic complications from greater than 1500 procedures (less than 0.3%).[21] The neurologic complications of kyphoplasty have generally occurred early in the experience of the physicians and have involved improper tool placement. One patient sustained an anterior cord syndrome from loss of collateral blood supply. This patient had a severely collapsed vertebra with the end plate below the pedicles. Needle placement was infrapedicular to avoid the disk space. Hemiparesis resulted in one patient when the needle was placed too far medial, causing spinal cord injury. Lower extremity weakness resulted in a third patient when PMMA was placed into the epidural space, and an epidural hematoma resulted in a fourth patient who had residual coagulopathy at the time of the procedure.

One patient developed significant postoperative ileus secondary to a large retroperitoneal hematoma that resulted from a perioperative coagulopathy due to Coumadin usage. Also reported was hypoxia and fever in a patient with a venous leak of PMMA that was injected in a low-viscosity state.

There have been no reported complications caused by inflation of the balloon.

Three patients have had perioperative pulmonary edema related to excessive intraoperative fluid administration, and there are two reported cases of postoperative myocardial infarction.

■ Kyphoplasty Complication Avoidance

As with vertebroplasty, appropriate patient selection and meticulous surgical technique are key in avoiding the potential complications.

Infection, solid metastatic tumor, and posterior wall breach or fracture with canal intrusion and disk herniation are contraindications to the procedure. Similarly, all coagulopathies should be corrected prior to the procedure. Perhaps the key difference for kyphoplasty is its utility in the treatment of acute fractures. Because cement is injected into a preformed void of known volume under low pressure in a highly viscous state, cement leakage is much less likely to occur. Thus kyphoplasty may be used to treat acute vertebral compression fractures.

Only those physicians with special training in image-guided and balloon inflation spinal procedures should consider performing kyphoplasty. Completion of a course run by expert faculty that includes thorough, hands on, cadaver experience is a prerequisite for performing this technique. Frequent use of anteroposterior and lateral imaging during tool placement, balloon reduction, and cavity fill will reduce the risk of complications related to cement leakage. An additional advantage of kyphoplasty during the PMMA injection phase is that, after balloon inflation, the volume of cement that will be injected is known, thus adding a further margin of safety.

Slow, gradual balloon inflation under anteroposterior and lateral image guidance will prevent vertebral wall or end-plate fracture.

As with vertebroplasty, careful attention to patient positioning and gentle technique will avoid rib fractures and pressure ulcerations. Antibiotics can be used in the cement to help reduce the risk of infection.

■ Management of Complications Related to Vertebroplasty and Kyphoplasty

Epidural Cement Leakage

If cement is found to have extravasated into the spinal canal, the patient should be awakened from general anesthesia and neurologic status should be assessed. If a new neurologic deficit indicating spinal cord injury or cauda equina syndrome is present, then decompression is mandated. The decision to approach the decompression from anterior or posterior depends on many variables, including thoracic or lumbar level, location of the cement, and the ability of the patient to withstand a thoracotomy. If no neurologic deficit exists, then the patient can be observed closely for the development of such.

Foraminal Cement Leakage

This is unlikely to cause a profound neurologic deficit; however, radiculitis or mild weakness can result. If radiculopathy or pain does not resolve or progresses, then a posterior decompression is recommended.

Neurologic Deficit

If a patient is found to have significant neurologic deficit in the recovery room or on the ward postoperatively despite no intraoperative indication of cement leakage, two possibilities may exist. Either cement leakage was not properly assessed with biplanar imaging, or bleeding has resulted in an epidural hematoma. Blood work should be done immediately to assess and correct any coagulopathy. This should be followed by urgent imaging, which may include a myelogram CT or magnetic resonance imaging. If canal compromise is found, then decompression is mandated.

Cerebrospinal Fluid Leakage

If CSF is noted to be leaking from the needle or puncture site, the hole should be packed with Gelfoam and injection of PMMA abandoned on that side.

Hypoxia and hypotension from PMMA injection should be treated symptomatically with oxygen, fluid resuscitation, and appropriate pharmacological support. Embolization of PMMA to the lungs has been successfully treated with anticoagulation. The presence of infection, if it does not respond to systemic antibiotic, may require debridement with fusion and reconstruction.

REFERENCES

1. Weill A, Chiras J, Simon JM, Rose M, Sola-Martinez T, Enkauoa E. Spinal metastases: indications for and results of percutaneous injection of acrylic surgical cement. Radiology 1996;199:241–247
2. Cotton A, Dewatre F, Cortet B, et al. Percutaneous vertebroplasty for osteolytic metastases and myeloma: effects of the percentage of lesion filling and the leakage of methyl methacrylate at clinical follow-up. Radiology 1996;200:525–530
3. Deramond H, Deprieste C, Galibert P, Le Gars D. Percutaneous vertebroplasty with polymethylmethacrylate: techniques, indications, and results. Radiol Clin North Am 1998;36:533–546
4. Deramond H, Galibert P, Debussche-Depriester C, Pruvo JP, Heleg A, Hodes J. Percutaneous vertebroplasty with methylmethacrylate: technique, method, results. Radiology 1990;117(suppl):352
5. Padovani B, Kasriel O, Brunner P, Peretti-Viton P. Pulmonary embolism caused by acrylic cement: a rare complication of percutaneous vertebroplasty. AJNR Am J Neuroradiol 1999;20:375–377
6. Chiras J, Depriester C, Weill A, Sola-Martinez MT, Deramond H. [Percutaneous vertebral surgery: techniques and indications] (in French). J Neuroradiol 1997;24:45–59
7. Wenger M, Markwalder TM. Surgically controlled, transpedicular methyl methacrylate vertebroplasty with fluoroscopic guidance. Acta Neurochir (Wien) 1999;141:625–631
8. Moreland DB, Landi MK, Grand W. Techniques to avoid complications in percutaneous vertebroplasty. Presented at the 15th annual meeting of the North American Society, New Orleans, October 2000
9. Jensen ME, Evans AJ, Mathis JM, Kallmes DF, Cloft HJ, Dion JE. Percutaneous polymethylmethacrylate vertebroplasty in the treatment of osteoporotic vertebral body compression fractures: technical aspects. AJNR Am J Neuroradiol 1997;18:1897–1904
10. Cyteval C, Sarrabere MP, Roux JO, et al. Acute osteoporotic vertebral collapse: open study on percutaneous injection of acrylic surgical cement in 20 patients. AJR Am J Roentgenol 1999;173:1685–1690
11. Martin JB, Jean B, Sugui K, et al. Vertebroplasty: clinical experience and follow-up results. Bone 1999;25(2 suppl):11S–15S
12. Cortet B, Cotton A, Boutry N, et al. Percutaneous vertebroplasty in the treatment of osteoporotic compression fractures: an open prospective study. J Rheumatol 1999;26:2222–2228
13. Barr JD, Barr MS, Lemley TJ, McCann RM. Percutaneous vertebroplasty for pain relief and spinal stabilization. Spine 2000;25:923–928
14. Convery FR, Gunn DR, Hughes JD, Martin WE. The relative safety of polymethylmethacrylate: a controlled clinical study of randomly selected patients treated with Charnley and ring total hip replacements. J Bone Joint Surg 1975;57A:57–64
15. Phillips H, Cole PV, Letton AW. Cardiovascular effects of implanted acrylic bone cement. BMJ 1971;3:460–461
16. Peh WC, Gilula LA, Zeller D. Percutaneous vertebroplasty: a new technique for treatment of painful compression fractures. Mo Med 2001;98:97–102
17. Medical Device Report Listing FDA. www.CDRH.FDA.gov/MAUDE
18. Wong WO, Garfin SR, Reiley MA. Kyphoplasty and vertebroplasty. J Women's Imaging 2000;2:117
19. Belkoff SM, Mathis JM, Fenton DC, et al. An ex vivo biomechanical evaluation of an inflatable bone tamp used in the treatment of compression fracture. Spine 2001;26:151–156
20. Lieberman IH, Dudeney S, Reinhardt MK, et al. Initial outcome and efficacy of "kyphoplasty" in the treatment of painful osteoporotic vertebral compression fractures. Spine 2001;26:1631–1638
21. Garfin SR, Yuan HA, Reiley MA. New technologies in spine: kyphoplasty and vertebroplasty for the treatment of painful osteoporotic compression fractures. Spine 2001;26:1511–1515

11

Vertebroplasty and Kyphoplasty: Advantages and Disadvantages

FRANK M. PHILLIPS AND WADE H. WONG

Objectives: On completion of this chapter, the reader should be able to discuss management strategies to minimize the risk of complications following vertebroplasty or kyphoplasty.

Accreditation: The American Association of Neurological Surgeons is accredited by the Accreditation Council for Continuing Medical Education to sponsor continuing medical education for physicians.

Credit: The American Association of Neurological Surgeons designates this continuing medical education activity for a maximum of 15 credits in Category I of the Physician's Recognition Award of the American Medical Association.

The Home Study Examination is online at www.aans.org/education/books/vertebro.asp

Osteoporotic vertebral compression fractures (VCFs) are a leading cause of disability and morbidity in the elderly.[1,2] The consequences of these fractures include pain and, in many cases, progressive vertebral collapse with resultant spinal kyphosis. Osteoporotic VCFs have been shown to adversely affect quality of life, physical function, mental health, and survival.[2-4] These effects are related to the severity of the spinal deformity and are in part independent of pain.[2,3] Spinal kyphosis leads to physical deformity and may cause chronic mechanical back pain. In recent years, researchers have highlighted reduced quality of life, functional limitations, and impaired pulmonary function associated with osteoporotic VCFs and spinal deformity.[1,2,5-8] Leech et al[5] have reported a 9% decrease in pulmonary vital capacity for each thoracic vertebral fracture. Kyphosis can lead to reduced abdominal space with poor appetite and resultant nutritional problems.[2,9] By shifting the patient's center of gravity forward, kyphotic deformity not only increases the risk of additional fractures,[10] but also may lead to poor balance, which potentially increases the risk of accidental falls.[11,12] In addition to the morbidity associated with VCFs, a prospective study reported an increased mortality rate in older women with VCFs compared with age-matched controls.[13] The mortality rate was related to pulmonary problems and increased with the number of vertebra fractured.

The ideal surgical treatment of osteoporotic vertebral compression fractures should address both the fracture-related pain and the kyphotic deformity. This should be accomplished in a minimally invasive fashion without subjecting the patient to inordinate risks or excessive surgical trauma. Over the past decade, percutaneous vertebroplasty, involving the injection of polymethyl-methacrylate (PMMA) into a fractured vertebral body in an attempt to alleviate pain, has been popularized. Substantial pain relief has been reported in a majority of patients treated with vertebroplasty for osteopenic VCF.[14-22] Although effective at relieving vertebral fracture pain, vertebroplasty is not designed to address the associated sagittal plane deformity. Kyphoplasty involves the penetration of the vertebral body with a trocar followed by insertion of an inflatable balloon tamp. Inflation of the balloon tamp restores the vertebral body back toward its original height, while creating a cavity to be filled with bone void filler. This technique was first performed in 1998, and early results of kyphoplasty suggest significant pain relief as well as the ability to improve height of the collapsed vertebral body.[23-28]

PMMA has been the most common bone void filler used in both vertebroplasty and kyphoplasty. This acrylic cement typically has been used for the fixation of metal and plastic joint replacements and for the fixation of pathologic fractures.[29,30] When used to treat vertebral

TABLE 11–1 Characteristics of Vertebroplasty and Kyphoplasty

Vertebroplasty	Kyphoplasty
Good pain relief	Good pain relief
Simple, quick, inexpensive	Equipment cost and time
Local anesthesia	Local or general anesthesia
Lower viscosity cement	Higher viscosity "doughy" cement
Extravertebral cement leakage: =70%	Extravertebral cement leakage: <10%
No impact on kyphosis	Reduces kyphosis

compression fractures, PMMA is usually modified (for example, addition of more barium sulfate, addition of antibiotics, alteration of monomer to powder ratio) in part, to attain a viscosity that would allow percutaneous insertion into vertebrae while minimizing the risk of extravertebral leaks. In April 2004 the United States Food and Drug Administration (FDA) approved a formulation of PMMA for use in vertebroplasty and kyphoplasty procedures.

Both vertebroplasty and kyphoplasty appear to be useful techniques in the management of osteopenic vertebral fractures. Discussion of the relative merits of these procedures focuses on the specific goals of each procedure as well as the safety and effectiveness of the procedure in accomplishing these goals (Table **11–1**).

■ Vertebroplasty

Suggested indications for vertebroplasty include stabilization of painful osteoporotic vertebral fractures, painful vertebra due to osteolytic metastases or multiple myeloma, Kummell's disease, and painful vertebral hemangioma. Vertebroplasty has been performed widely with relatively few major complications reported.[14–17,19,20,22] Reports on the outcome for vertebroplasty have suggested that most patients experience partial or complete pain relief within 72 hours of the procedure.[14,16,19,22,31–36] Overall, 60 to 100% of patients reported in the literature noted decreased pain after vertebroplasty.[19,34] In addition to decreased pain, improved functional levels and reduced analgesic medication requirements have been reported.[22,34,37–40] Zoarski et al[41] used the Musculoskeletal Outcomes Data Evaluation and Management Scale (MODEMS) administered before and at 2 weeks after vertebroplasty in 30 patients. Significant improvement in all four modules of the MODEMS (treatment score, pain and disability, physical function, mental function) was demonstrated. Grados et al[20] reported longer-term follow-up of a cohort of patients with osteoporotic VCFs treated with vertebroplasty. Of 40 patients treated with vertebroplasty, 25 were available for follow-up at a mean of 48 months. Pain decreased from a mean of 80 mm

before vertebroplasty to 37 mm after 1 month. These results remained stable over time, with a pain score of 34 mm at final follow-up (mean 48 months). Published reports have noted a low complication rate for vertebroplasty, with most complications resulting from extravertebral cement leakage causing spinal cord or nerve root compression or pulmonary embolism.[14,16,19,22,31–36]

Complications with vertebroplasty largely relate to extravertebral cement extravasation during the procedure. During vertebroplasty, bone cement is injected into the fractured vertebral body. The cement tends to be "runny" to permit injection into cancellous bone through a narrow-gauge needle. Cement may leak out of the vertebral body directly through deficiencies in the vertebral body cortex or via the venous system. If PMMA extravasates outside of the vertebral body, complications related to mechanical or thermal injury of adjacent anatomic structures may occur. The risk of local cement leakage is likely affected by cement injection pressure and cement viscosity, as well as the ability of the bone, particularly the vertebral body cortex, to resist cement leakage. Proponents of vertebroplasty have recommended discontinuing cement injection once cement extravasation beyond the vertebral body is seen.

In addition to the risks of local cement leakage, occasional cardiovascular collapse has been associated with the surgical use of PMMA during arthroplasty surgery.[42–45] It has been hypothesized that pressurization of PMMA into cancellous bone predisposes to embolization of cement, methylmethacrylate monomer, and bone marrow contents to the lungs with resulting adverse cardiopulmonary sequelae.[42–44,46] This is certainly a cause for concern during vertebral augmentation procedures when high-pressure PMMA injection into vertebral bodies is performed.

Although extravertebral cement extravasation is commonly seen with vertebroplasty, infrequent clinical sequelae of the leakage have been reported. Cortet et al[15] reported extravertebral cement in 13 of 20 vertebrae (65%) treated with vertebroplasty for osteoporotic fractures. Cement leakage into the paravertebral soft tissue occurred in six patients, into the peridural space in three patients, into the disk space in three patients, and into the lumbar venous plexus in one patient. Cyteval et al[16] noted extravertebral cement in eight of 20 patients (40%) after vertebroplasty, with leakage into the intervertebral disk in five patients, into the neural foramen in two patients, and into the lumbar venous plexus in one patient. Deramond et al[17] reported radiculopathy in 4% of patients undergoing vertebroplasty, likely related to intraforaminal cement leakage. With vertebroplasty to treat painful osteolytic metastases or multiple myeloma, Cortet et al[14] reported extravertebral cement leakage in 29 of 37 patients (79%). In addition to the risk of local cement extravasation, radiographic evidence of PMMA

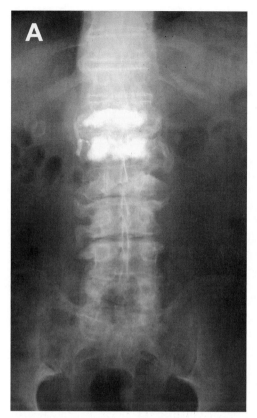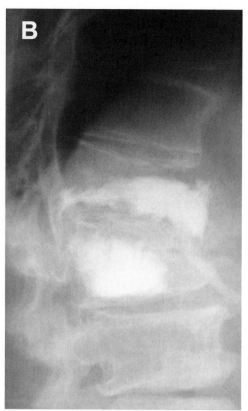

FIGURE 11–1 A 78-year-old man with L2 and L3 vertebral compression fracture treated with vertebroplasty 3 months after fracture. **(A)** Postoperative anteroposterior radiograph. **(B)** Postoperative lateral radiograph. (From Phillips FM. Minimally invasive treatments of osteoporotic vertebral compression fractures. Spine 2003;28(15S):S45–53, with permission.)

pulmonary embolism after vertebroplasty has been reported.[20,22,47–49]

Traditionally, vertebroplasty makes no attempt to correct kyphosis, and therefore it does not influence sagittal plane deformity (Fig. **11–1**). Consequently, vertebroplasty usually does not afford the opportunity of impacting the effects of kyphosis on health. Recent reports suggest that some vertebral body height restoration can be achieved in vertebroplasty procedures with or without postural reduction if the VCF is characterized by an intravertebral cleft.[50–54] Further research is needed to determine how widespread this phenomenon is, and controlled studies are warranted to compare height restoration and complication rates associated with vertebroplasty with those of kyphoplasty, which is performed under more controlled conditions.

Accurate clinical diagnosis and workup are critical to the success of vertebral augmentation procedures. Elderly patients with osteoporotic VCFs may have multiple sources of back pain. Clinical expertise is necessary to determine whether any back pain is related to the VCF seen on radiographic studies. Additionally, in the setting of back pain with multiple fractures visualized on radiographs, it can be difficult to determine which, if any, of the fractures require treatment. These treatment decisions require in-depth knowledge of spinal fracture management. If a nonspine surgeon is to perform vertebroplasty, it is essential to have a spinal surgeon available to treat potential complications of the procedure. PMMA in the epidural space causing symptomatic neural compression has been reported and may require urgent surgical decompression.[17,55] Where circumstances allow, a team approach to vertebroplasty involving both an invasive neuroradiologist and a spinal surgeon is optimal.

On the other hand, vertebroplasty is a less expensive procedure than kyphoplasty. The equipment required for vertebroplasty is simple and inexpensive when compared with the kyphoplasty tools. Vertebroplasty is usually performed in a fluoroscopy suite under local anesthesia, thereby eliminating costs that might be incurred in the operating room. Because fewer steps are involved the procedure generally takes less time than kyphoplasty. In addition, fluoroscopy units in an interventional radiology suite are typically superior to the portable units used in most operating rooms, resulting in better quality of images and improved speed of operation. Although performing these procedures in an outpatient setting in the radiology suite is desirable and may be cost-saving, adequate resuscitative and postprocedural patient monitoring capabilities must be readily available.

■ Kyphoplasty

Kyphoplasty involves percutaneous placement of an inflatable balloon tamp (IBT) into a fractured vertebral body. Balloon tamp inflation results in a cavity being created within the vertebral body as well as elevation of the depressed vertebral body end plate. These IBT effects are an attempt to address the shortcomings of vertebroplasty; that is, high rates of cement leakage and inability to correct fracture deformity (Fig. 11–2). As the balloon tamp is inflated in the fractured vertebral body, cancellous bone is pushed away from the balloon, creating a cavity surrounded by compacted cancellous bone.[56–58] The creation of an intravertebral cavity may decrease the potential for cement leakage by allowing for low-pressure, controlled placement of "doughy" cement into the cavity and by creating a dam effect by densely compacting bone around the cavity.

Wong et al[28] reported on 85 patients treated with kyphoplasty, one of whom had a presumed cement embolus to the lungs. This occurred early in the kyphoplasty experience when highly runny cement was used. As experience with kyphoplasty has been gained, it has become apparent that the intravertebral cavity created by the IBT allows for placement of more viscous, partially cured cement. Lieberman et al[25] reported on 70 fractured vertebral bodies treated with kyphoplasty and noted extravertebral cement leakage in 8.6% of

levels treated. Cement leakage was epidural at one level, into the disk space at two levels, and into the paravertebral soft tissues at three levels. None of the leaks had any adverse clinical consequences. Similarly, Ledlie and Renfro[24] reported asymptomatic cement leakage in 9% (12/133) of treated fractures, and Phillips et al[26] reported clinically insignificant cement leakage in 9.8% (6/61) of cases, including four leaks to the adjacent intervertebral disk, one leak anterior to the treated level, and one case with leaks to both the intervertebral disk and anterior regions. In a cadaver study, Belkoff et al[59] reported extravertebral cement leakage in five of eight human vertebral bodies treated with vertebroplasty, with no cement leakage seen in vertebrae treated with kyphoplasty. In addition, Phillips et al[58] have completed a study comparing contrast spread after intravertebral injection at the time of vertebroplasty and kyphoplasty. With contrast injections during kyphoplasty, contrast is seen to fill the cavity created by the IBT with occasional extravertebral leakage. In vertebroplasty injections, leakage of contrast outside of the vertebral bodies invariably occurs with frequent fill of the inferior vena cava and epidural vessels.

In the series of Wong et al,[28] 80 of 85 patients reported good to excellent pain relief after kyphoplasty. Lieberman et al[25] reported highly significant improvement in physical function, role physical, vitality, mental health, and social function scores of the SF-36 questionnaire

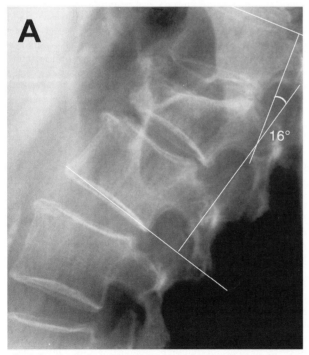
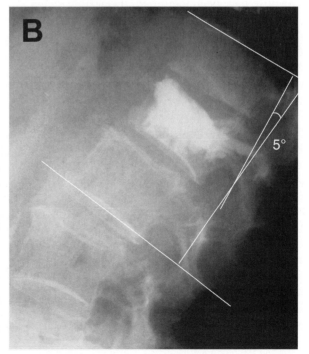

FIGURE 11–2 A 73-year-old woman with L1 vertebral compression fracture treated with kyphoplasty 6 weeks after fracture. The focal kyphosis was corrected from 16 to 5 degrees. **(A)** Preoperative lateral radiograph. **(B)** Postoperative lateral radiograph. (From Phillips FM. Minimally invasive treatments of osteoporotic vertebral compression fractures. Spine 2003; 28(15S):S45–53, with permission.)

after kyphoplasty. Ledlie and Renfro[24] reported rapid reduction in pain and improvement in activity levels in their cohort of 96 patients. In addition to pain relief, kyphoplasty also affords the opportunity to restore vertebral body height and thereby improve spinal sagittal balance. Wong et al[28] noted that anterior vertebral body height increased from 79% ± 22% to 99% ± 13% of calculated normal anterior vertebral body height after kyphoplasty. Lieberman et al[25] reported at least 10% height restoration in 70% of 70 fractured vertebrae treated with kyphoplasty. In those patients in whom the vertebral fractures could be reduced by kyphoplasty, vertebral height was increased by a mean of 46.8%. Ledlie and Renfro observed anterior and midline vertebral body height increases after kyphoplasty that were stable through 1-year follow-up. The height was ~65% preoperatively and 90% postoperatively for anterior and midline measurements for this series of patients. In addition, Phillips et al[26] reported on a series of 29 patients (61 VCFs) treated with kyphoplasty. In those patients in whom fracture reduction occurred, local kyphosis was improved by a mean of 14 degrees. The ability to reduce kyphosis in a controlled manner is a significant advantage of kyphoplasty over vertebroplasty.

A frustration with kyphoplasty has been the unpredictability of fracture reduction with this technique. As fracture healing progresses, the IBT is less likely to effect a fracture reduction. To date, no specific clinical or radiographic parameters that accurately predict the ability to reduce a fracture have been identified. It certainly seems plausible that earlier treatment of the fracture increases the likelihood of IBT-mediated fracture reduction.

Although kyphoplasty may offer potential clinical advantages over vertebroplasty, kyphoplasty is a more expensive procedure. Kyphoplasty requires the use of specialized surgical instruments and has typically been performed in the operating room, although one of the authors (W.H.W.) performs kyphoplasty in the interventional radiology suite. Long-term studies are required to determine whether correction of spinal deformity obtained with kyphoplasty will reduce long-term medical expenses, and as a result offset the increased surgical cost of kyphoplasty. Both kyphoplasty and vertebroplasty are useful techniques for spine physicians and their patients. Further studies are required to determine the relative merits of both procedures as well as the precise role for these procedures in managing patients with osteopenic vertebral compression fractures.

REFERENCES

1. Lyles KW, Gold DT, Shipp KM, Pieper CF, Martinez S, Mulhausen PL. Association of osteoporotic vertebral compression fractures with impaired functional status. Am J Med 1993;94:595–601
2. Silverman SL. The clinical consequences of vertebral compression fracture. Bone 1992;13(suppl 2):S27–S31
3. Gold DT. The clinical impact of vertebral fractures: quality of life in women with osteoporosis. Bone 1996;18:185S–189S
4. Gold DT, Lyles KW. Fractures: effects on quality of life. In: Rosen CJ, Glowacki J, Bilezikian JP, eds. The Aging Skeleton. San Diego: Academic Press, 1999:632
5. Leech JA, Dulberg C, Kellie S, Pattee L, Gay J. Relationship of lung function to severity of osteoporosis in women. Am Rev Respir Dis 1990;141:68–71
6. Leidig G, Minne HW, Sauer P, et al. A study of complaints and their relation to vertebral destruction in patients with osteoporosis. Bone Miner 1990;8:217–229
7. Pluijm SM, Tromp AM, Smit JH, Deeg DJ, Lips P. Consequences of vertebral deformities in older men and women. J Bone Miner Res 2000;15:1564–1572
8. Schlaich C, Minne HW, Bruckner T, et al. Reduced pulmonary function in patients with spinal osteoporotic fractures. Osteoporos Int 1998;8:261–267
9. Ross PD, Davis JW, Epstein RS, Wasnich RD. Pain and disability associated with new vertebral fractures and other spinal conditions. J Clin Epidemiol 1994;47:231–239
10. Lindsay R, Silverman SL, Cooper C, et al. Risk of new vertebral fracture in the year following a fracture. JAMA 2001;285:320–323
11. Keller TS, Harrison DE, Colloca CJ, Harrison DD, Janik TJ. Prediction of osteoporotic spinal deformity. Spine 2003;28:455–462
12. White AA III, Panjabi MM, Thomas CL. The clinical biomechanics of kyphotic deformities. Clin Orthop 1977;128:8–17
13. Kado DM, Browner WS, Palermo L, Nevitt MC, Genant HK, Cummings SR. Vertebral fractures and mortality in older women: a prospective study. Arch Intern Med 1999;159:1215–1220
14. Cortet B, Cotten A, Boutry N, et al. Percutaneous vertebroplasty in the treatment of osteoporotic vertebral compression fractures: an open prospective study. J Rheumatol 1999;26:2222–2228
15. Cortet B, Cotten A, Boutry N, et al. Percutaneous vertebroplasty in patients with osteolytic metastases or multiple myeloma. Rev Rhum Engl Ed 1997;64:177–183
16. Cyteval C, Sarrabere MP, Roux JO, et al. Acute osteoporotic vertebral collapse: open study on percutaneous injection of acrylic surgical cement in 20 patients. AJR Am J Roentgenol 1999;173:1685–1690
17. Deramond H, Depriester C, Galibert P, Le Gars D. Percutaneous vertebroplasty with polymethylmethacrylate: technique, indications, and results. Radiol Clin North Am 1998;36:533–546
18. Evans AJ, Jensen ME, Kip KE, et al. Vertebral compression fractures: pain reduction and improvement in functional mobility after percutaneous polymethylmethacrylate vertebroplasty retrospective report of 245 cases. Radiology 2003;226:366–372
19. Gangi A, Kastler BA, Dietemann JL. Percutaneous vertebroplasty guided by a combination of CT and fluoroscopy. AJNR Am J Neuroradiol 1994;15:83–86
20. Grados F, Depriester C, Cayrolle G, Hardy N, Deramond H, Fardellone P. Long-term observations of vertebral osteoporotic fractures treated by percutaneous vertebroplasty. Rheumatology (Oxf) 2000;39:1410–1414
21. Hodler J, Peck D, Gilula LA. Midterm outcome after vertebroplasty: predictive value of technical and patient-related factors. Radiology 2003;227:662–668
22. Jensen ME, Evans AJ, Mathis JM, Kallmes DF, Cloft HJ, Dion JE. Percutaneous polymethylmethacrylate vertebroplasty in the treatment of osteoporotic vertebral body compression fractures: technical aspects. AJNR Am J Neuroradiol 1997;18:1897–1904
23. Dudeney S, Lieberman IH, Reinhardt MK, Hussein M. Kyphoplasty in the treatment of osteolytic vertebral compression fractures as a result of multiple myeloma. J Clin Oncol 2002;20:2382–2387
24. Ledlie JT, Renfro M. Balloon kyphoplasty: one-year outcomes in vertebral body height restoration, chronic pain, and activity levels. J Neurosurg Spine 2003;98:36–42

25. Lieberman IH, Dudeney S, Reinhardt MK, Bell G. Initial outcome and efficacy of "kyphoplasty" in the treatment of painful osteoporotic vertebral compression fractures. Spine 2001;26:1631–1638

26. Phillips FM, Ho E, Campbell-Hupp M, McNally T, Todd Wetzel F, Gupta P. Early radiographic and clinical results of balloon kyphoplasty for the treatment of osteoporotic vertebral compression fractures. Spine 2003;28:2260–2265

27. Theodorou DJ, Wong WH, Duncan TD, Garfin SR, Theodorou SJ, Stoll T. Percutaneous Balloon Kyphoplasty: Initial Experience with the Application of a Novel Procedure for the Correction of Spinal Deformity Associated with Vertebral Compression Fractures. San Francisco: American Academy of Orthopaedic Surgeons, 2001

28. Wong WH, Reiley MA, Garfin SR. Vertebroplasty/kyphoplasty. J Women's Imaging 2000;2:117–124

29. Bauer TW, Schils J. The pathology of total joint arthroplasty. I. Mechanisms of implant fixation. Skeletal Radiol 1999; 28:423–432

30. Jang JS, Lee SH, Rhee CH, Lee SH. Polymethylmethacrylate-augmented screw fixation for stabilization in metastatic spinal tumors. Technical note. J Neurosurg Spine 2002;96:131–134

31. Chiras J, Depriester C, Weill A, Sola-Martinez MT, Deramond H. [Percutaneous vertebral surgery. Techniques and indications] (in French). J Neuroradiol 1997;24:45–59

32. Hardouin P, Grados F, Cotten A, Cortet B. Should percutaneous vertebroplasty be used to treat osteoporotic fractures? An update. Joint Bone Spine 2001;68:216–221

33. Lapras C, Mottolese C, Deruty R, Lapras C Jr, Remond J, Duquesnel J. [Percutaneous injection of methyl-methacrylate in osteoporosis and severe vertebral osteolysis (Galibert's technique)] (in French). Ann Chir 1989;43:371–376

34. Mathis JM, Petri M, Naff N. Percutaneous vertebroplasty treatment of steroid-induced osteoporotic compression fractures. Arthritis Rheum 1998;41:171–175

35. Rapado A. General management of vertebral fractures. Bone 1996;18:191S–196S

36. Watts NB, Harris ST, Genant HK. Treatment of painful osteoporotic vertebral fractures with percutaneous vertebroplasty or kyphoplasty. Osteoporos Int 2001;12:429–437

37. Amar AP, Larsen DW, Esnaashari N, Albuquerque FC, Lavine SD, Teitelbaum GP. Percutaneous transpedicular polymethylmethacrylate vertebroplasty for the treatment of spinal compression fractures. Neurosurgery 2001;49:1105–1114; discussion 1114–1105

38. Kim AK, Jensen ME, Dion JE, Schweickert PA, Kaufmann TJ, Kallmes DF. Unilateral transpedicular percutaneous vertebroplasty: initial experience. Radiology 2002;222:737–741

39. Martin JB, Jean B, Sugiu K, et al. Vertebroplasty: clinical experience and follow-up results. Bone 1999;25:11S–15S

40. Tsou IY, Goh PY, Peh WC, Goh LA, Chee TS. Percutaneous vertebroplasty in the management of osteoporotic vertebral compression fractures: initial experience. Ann Acad Med Singapore 2002;31:15–20

41. Zoarski GH, Snow P, Olan WJ, et al. Percutaneous vertebroplasty for osteoporotic compression fractures: quantitative prospective evaluation of long-term outcomes. J Vasc Intervent Radiol 2002; 13:139–148

42. Markel DC, Femino JE, Farkas P, Markel SF. Analysis of lower extremity embolic material after total knee arthroplasty in a canine model. J Arthroplasty 1999;14:227–232

43. Orsini EC, Byrick RJ, Mullen JB, Kay JC, Waddell JP. Cardiopulmonary function and pulmonary microemboli during arthroplasty using cemented or non-cemented components: the role of intramedullary pressure. J Bone Joint Surg Am 1987;69:822–832

44. Pinto PW. Cardiovascular collapse associated with the use of methylmethacrylate. AANA J 1993;61:613–616

45. Pitto RP, Blunk J, Kossler M. Transesophageal echocardiography and clinical features of fat embolism during cemented total hip arthroplasty: a randomized study in patients with a femoral neck fracture. Arch Orthop Trauma Surg 2000;120:53–58

46. Rudigier JF, Ritter G. Pathogenesis of circulatory reactions triggered by nervous reflexes during the implantation of bone cements. Res Exp Med (Berl) 1983;183:77–94

47. Chen HL, Wong CS, Ho ST, Chang FL, Hsu CH, Wu CT. A lethal pulmonary embolism during percutaneous vertebroplasty. Anesth Analg 2002;95:1060–1062

48. Gangi A, Dietemann JL, Guth S, Steib JP, Roy C. Computed tomography (CT) and fluoroscopy-guided vertebroplasty: results and complications in 187 patients. Semin Intervent Radiol 1999; 16:137–142

49. Padovani B, Kasriel O, Brunner P, Peretti-Viton P. Pulmonary embolism caused by acrylic cement: a rare complication of percutaneous vertebroplasty. AJNR Am J Neuroradiol 1999;20:375–377

50. Hiwatashi A, Moritani T, Numaguchi Y, Westesson PL. Increase in vertebral body height after vertebroplasty. AJNR Am J Neuroradiol 2003;24:185–189

51. McKiernan F, Jensen R, Faciszewski T. The dynamic mobility of vertebral compression fractures. J Bone Miner Res 2003;18: 24–29

52. Nakano M, Hirano N, Matsuura K, et al. Percutaneous transpedicular vertebroplasty with calcium phosphate cement in the treatment of osteoporotic vertebral compression and burst fractures. J Neurosurg 2002;97:287–293

53. Peh WC, Gelbart MS, Gilula LA, Peck DD. Percutaneous vertebroplasty: treatment of painful vertebral compression fractures with intraosseous vacuum phenomena. AJR Am J Roentgenol 2003; 180:1411–1417

54. Teng MM, Wei CJ, Wei LC, et al. Kyphosis correction and height restoration effects of percutaneous vertebroplasty. AJNR Am J Neuroradiol 2003;24:1893–1900

55. Cotten A, Dewatre F, Cortet B, et al. Percutaneous vertebroplasty for osteolytic metastases and myeloma: effects of the percentage of lesion filling and the leakage of methyl methacrylate at clinical follow-up. Radiology 1996;200:525–530

56. Garfin SR, Yuan HA, Reiley MA. New technologies in spine: kyphoplasty and vertebroplasty for the treatment of painful osteoporotic compression fractures. Spine 2001;26:1511–1515

57. Lane JM, Johnson CE, Khan SN, Girardi FP, Cammisa FP Jr. Minimally invasive options for the treatment of osteoporotic vertebral compression fractures. Orthop Clin North Am 2002;33:431–438, viii.

58. Phillips FM, Todd Wetzel F, Lieberman I, Campbell-Hupp M. An in vivo comparison of the potential for extravertebral cement leak after vertebroplasty and kyphoplasty. Spine 2002;27:2173–2178; discussion 2178–2179

59. Belkoff SM, Mathis JM, Fenton DC, Scribner RM, Reiley ME, Talmadge K. An ex vivo biomechanical evaluation of an inflatable bone tamp used in the treatment of compression fracture. Spine 2001;26:151–156

12

Vertebroplasty and Kyphoplasty: The Radiologist's Perspective

JOHN M. MATHIS

Objectives: On completion of this chapter, the reader should be able to compare and contrast the techniques of vertebroplasty and kyphoplasty in terms of indications, patient selection criteria, and complications.

Accreditation: The American Association of Neurological Surgeons is accredited by the Accreditation Council for Continuing Medical Education to sponsor continuing medical education for physicians.

Credit: The American Association of Neurological Surgeons designates this continuing medical education activity for a maximum of 15 credits in Category I of the Physician's Recognition Award of the American Medical Association.

The Home Study Examination is online at www.aans.org/education/books/vertebro.asp

When one sees the phrase *vertebroplasty* vs. *kyphoplasty*, we generally think of competitive procedures and, similarly, competitive groups of operative physicians. However, having had the opportunity to be involved in the development and introduction of percutaneous vertebroplasty (PV) and kyphoplasty (KP) in the United States,[1–21] it is my opinion that both offer substantial benefit and promise. The real hurdles now are to establish the appropriate differential indications, advantages, and shortcomings of each procedure. We must then select the appropriate method of therapy to maximally benefit our patients. This chapter looks at a comparison of these two techniques based on accumulated data rather than marketing claims.

■ History

By reviewing the history of the development of each procedure, we can better understand how a competitive environment has arisen between the procedures and many of the physicians using them.

PV had its inception in France in 1984,[22,23] where it was found useful for the treatment of pain associated with vertebral injury resulting from benign and malignant tumors, and subsequently, osteoporotic compression fractures. The technique spread to the United States in the early 1990s with our first report appearing in 1997.[10]

Since this early work, multiple papers have appeared describing the biomechanical effects of PV[11–20] and the clinical results of this therapy for the pain resulting from vertebral compression fractures (VCFs).[1–3,10,22,24–28] There has never been a prospective, randomized series comparing PV to alternative therapy. Nevertheless, essentially all reports have been exceedingly positive, showing substantial improvement in the patient's pain and the ability to resume activities of daily living. The effects of therapy have been durable, and clinical complications uncommon in the hands of experienced operators treating benign compression fractures (most series seem to report a higher risk of complications in patients with malignant disease). PV was first performed in Europe and the United States by neuroradiologists, and radiologists remain the most frequent users of this procedure at the time of this writing.

The idea of combining the pain relief of PV with a device that could also restore vertebral height was conceived by an orthopedic surgeon, Mark Reiley, who subsequently starting the device company Kyphon. The initial biomechanical investigations of the Kyphon device were performed as a combined effort by the developing orthopedic surgeon and the author.[15–17] The device was subsequently approved by the Food and Drug Administration (FDA) (on a 510K) as a "bone tamp." A randomized clinical trial (KP versus conservative medical therapy)

Mathis JM, Ortiz AO, Zoarski GH. Vertebroplasty versus kyphoplasty: a comparison and contrast. AJNR Am J Neuroradiol. 2004;25:840–845.

was attempted, but patient entry was slow and the idea ultimately abandoned in favor of a clinical registry tabulating the results of patients treated with KP. Therefore, this procedure, like PV, has not been tested by a comparison trial with conservative therapy. Clinical reports using KP are few, with the first peer-reviewed report available in 2001.[29] The authors found pain relief similar to that reported with PV and claimed no complications related to the procedure. Though there were no complications related to cement leaks, there was a 10% complication rate (3.3% major due to perioperative MI, and 6.6% minor due to rib fractures). Height restoration was enthusiastically reported by the authors, but analysis of their data reveals that the average height gained per vertebra treated is only ~3 mm (or slightly over 0.1 inch). This leaves open for argument the effectiveness of the device for predictably restoring vertebral height.

Early reports and discussions concerning the device were usually positive in the orthopedic community but negative among many radiologists, who were using PV but not KP. This initial difference of opinion has only increased as time has gone on. Currently, spinal surgeons perform the majority of KPs with a minority performed in the radiology community. This has been the primary source of the growing competition between the two groups of physicians and procedures. Unfortunately, this situation has been compounded by Kyphon limiting the access to the KP device mainly to orthopedic surgeons.

■ Jargon Versus Reality

It seems that most physicians agree that both PV and KP relieve the pain associated with vertebral compression fractures effectively and with similar results. This would seem intuitive, as KP employs the same vertebral stabilization technique used in PV, the introduction of bone cement into a compromised vertebra. KP has been referred to as "balloon-assisted PV."[30] Biomechanical data comparing the stabilizing effects created by PV and KP show similar results.[17]

Unfortunately, this reality has been blurred by the jargon. Purveyors of each procedure claim particular advantages over the other. One item of contention is the claim of the kyphoplasty group is that KP allows cement to be injected into a cavity (created by the bone tamp) at low-pressure which results in a lower likelihood of cement leak. This did not prevent a 8.6% cement leak rate reported by Lieberman et al.[29] Additionally, two independent labs have measured and reported the actual pressure in the vertebra during cement injections for both PV and KP and found no difference.[31,32] Also, to actually get biomechanical reinforcement of a fractured vertebra with KP, one must slightly overfill the void created by the bone tamp or recompression will immediately occur. This over-

filling would intuitively seem to require the same pressure necessary to fill a vertebra during PV as cement must be pushed into the intra-trabecular space, and therefore one would assume that similar final pressures are achieved during cement filling in both procedures. Lieberman's 8.5% asymptomatic cement leak is similar to that usually seen in my practice with PV (in over 1500 cases).

Both procedures are capable of, and have resulted in, severe complications due to cement leaks as are shown in the examples in Fig. 12–1. Indeed, Nussbaum et al reported on complications compiled by the FDA Maude website and found a similar death rate for both procedures (approximately 1/50,000 patients) and a 30 time higher permanent neurologic complication rate with KP than with PV (per patient procedure).[33] This difference is huge and may correlate with the added complexity of KP compared to PV. It certainly does not substantiate the marketing claims of reduced complications with KP.

An additional point of controversy revolves around the capability of KP to reliably produce height restoration in fractured and compressed vertebral bodies. Biomechanical evaluations by Belkoff et al[15] reported significant height restoration with KP compared with PV. However, their investigation looked only at vertebra that had a maximal height loss of 3 to 6 mm. KP did do a better job at restoring height in this situation of minimal compression. Unfortunately, no in vitro investigations are available that determine if this effect can be achieved when vertebra are more severely compressed. Indeed, Lieberman et al's[29] data (showing an average height restoration of only 3 mm per vertebra treated) suggest that KP may have a limited effect at height restoration in many patients. Alternatively, this limited clinical result could have resulted from poor patient selection. Many of Lieberman et al's patients were treated relatively late after fracture (average duration of symptoms was 5.9 months), and many could have experienced partial fracture healing prior to KP. No clinical trials are available that help us select those patients who will predictably get maximal height restoration using KP.

Initially, uses of PV did not look at height gain during this procedure. However, claims made by the marketers of KP spurred this investigation. Hiwatashi et al reported an average height restoration with PV of 2.2 mm (not substantially different from Lieberman's 3.0 mm).[34] McKeirnan et al found that vertebral height could be completely restored (100% of original height) in those vertebral that showed mobility during positioning for PV. Their absolute increase for these vertebra was 8.4 mm.[35] As there has been no comparison between KP and PV in a randomized trial, we are left to speculate that height restoration reported by KP may be largely that obtained simply by patient positioning as seen in PV. Reports also show significant kyphosis reduction with PV cases simply by positioning[36,37] (Fig. 12–2).

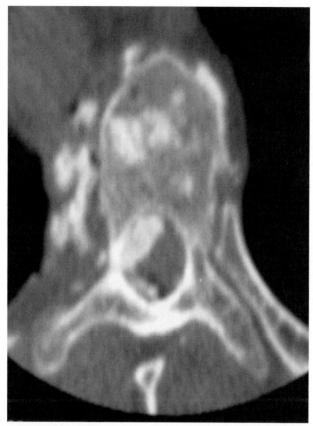

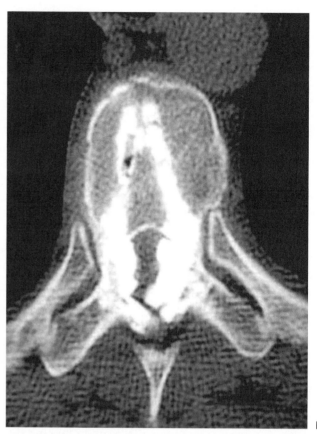

FIGURE 12–1 (A) Vertebroplasty complication. Computed tomography (CT) scan showing cement leaks into the spinal canal and paraspinous region after percutaneous vertebroplasty. This resulted in paraparesis of the lower extremities. **(B)** Kyphoplasty complication. CT scan showing large cement leaks into the spinal canal following a kyphoplasty procedure. This resulted in paraplegia of the lower extremities. (From JM Mathis. Percutaneous vertebroplasty. AJNR Am J Neuroradiol 2003;24:1697–1706; by permisson).

Pain relief seems less sensitive to "time from fracture" than height restoration. (As expected, pain relief in Lieberman et al's study was not adversely affected by treatment delay or height restoration achieved and was similar to that seen with PV.)

Some additional differences in the procedures involve the utilization of general anesthesia and hospitalization by surgeons versus conscious sedation (without the need for hospitalization) by radiologists. These differences seem to occur more because of the way each group works rather than by the requirement for either KP or PV. Certainly, there is no requirement for general anesthesia or hospitalization for either procedure in my practice.

Cost remains hugely different for the two procedures with the materials for KP approximately 10 times more expensive than the materials for PV. This may eventually be justified only if KP reliably produces height restoration in excess to that seen with PV. If significant height restoration can not be achieved, the medical market will ultimately dictate the frequency of utilization of each procedure.

■ Radiologist Perspective

Without doubt, both PV and KP need additional trials that conclusively establish the effectiveness of each against conservative medical therapy. A randomized comparison of PV and KP would also help establish patient selection criteria to better utilize these procedures to the patient's benefit. Until these data are available, we will continue to hear a considerable amount of jargon (and market hype) about the relative advantages of each procedure.

I believe that both procedures relieve pain and can be performed with acceptable complication rates (though it appears that the permanent neurologic complication rate for KP may be significantly higher than for PV). In my practice, I employ KP (with its inherent higher cost) only when I think that height restoration is very important due to severe kyphosis and the fracture is sufficiently acute to make the likelihood of height restoration substantial. I receive fractures that are referred at all time stages, including through the emergency department within hours of onset, but I tend to limit the performance

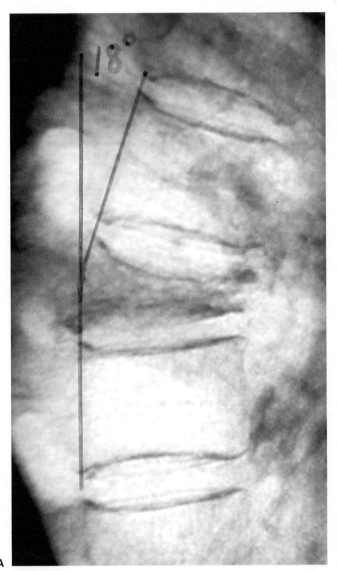

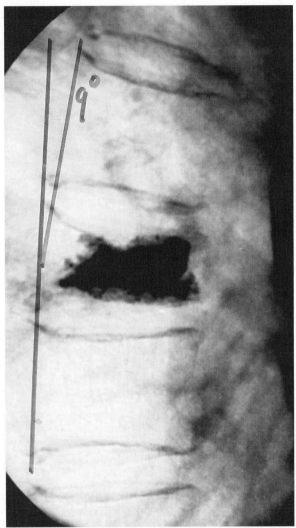

A   B

FIGURE 12–2 (A) Radiograph showing a severe compression fracture resulting in 18 degrees of kyphosis before PV. **(B)** Following PV, there is modest height gain, estimated at 3–4 mm, and a reduction in kyphosis to 9 degrees (50% change). (From JM Mathis. Percutaneous vertebroplasty. AJNR Am J Neuroradiol 2003;24:1697–1706; by permission).

of KP to patients whose fracture has occurred within the last 2 weeks. This criterion may be overly stringent, but as previously stated, no conclusive, alternative data are currently available for the selection of technique. Additionally, I have rarely seen substantial height restoration with KP in the majority of patients treated in my hospital and the literature offers little reliable criteria for determining who will achieve that height gain.

At the present time, I believe that both procedures should be available for use by every operator. I would hope that this would reduce the competition created by trying to overstate the marketed (but often unproven) advantages of one procedure versus another. Regardless of which procedure is chosen, safety depends on operator experience, excellent imaging equipment, and adequate

cement opacification. Most complications that occur with either procedure result from poor operator judgment or inadequate anatomic and cement visualization. Time and accumulated data will tell whether the promise of height restoration is actually achievable with KP. Until then, careful application of either procedure should successfully relieve the pain associated with vertebral compression injury.

REFERENCES

1. Mathis JM, Barr JD, Belkoff SM, et al. Percutaneous vertebroplasty: a developing standard of care for vertebral compression fractures. AJNR Am J Neuroradiol 2001;22:373–381
2. Mathis JM, Eckel TS, Belkoff SM, Deramond H. Percutaneous vertebroplasty: a therapeutic option for pain associated with vertebral

compression fracture. J Back Musculoskeletal Rehabil 1999; 12:1–7

3. Mathis JM, Petri M, Naff N. Percutaneous vertebroplasty treatment of steroid-induced osteoporotic compression fractures. Arthritis Rheum 1998;41:171–175

4. Mathis JM, Deramond H, Belkoff SM, eds. Percutaneous Vertebroplasty. New York: Springer-Verlag, 2002

5. Mathis JM. Procedural techniques and materials: tumors and osteoporotic fractures. In: Mathis JM, Deramond H, Belkoff SM, eds. Percutaneous Vertebroplasty. New York: Springer-Verlag, 2002: 81–107

6. Mathis JM, Belkoff SM, Deramond H. History and early development of percutaneous vertebroplasty. In: Mathis JM, Deramond H, Belkoff SM, eds. Percutaneous Vertebroplasty. New York: Springer-Verlag, 2002:1–5

7. Mathis JM, Belkoff SM, Deramond H. Future directions: challenges and research opportunities. In: Mathis JM, Deramond H, Belkoff SM, eds. Percutaneous Vertebroplasty. New York: Springer-Verlag, 2002:181–193

8. Mathis JM. Percutaneous vertebroplasty. In: Williams AL, Murtagh FR, eds. Handbook of Diagnostic and Therapeutic Spine Procedures. St. Louis: Mosby, 2002:153–166

9. Olan WJ, Mathis JM. Starting a clinical practice. In: Mathis JM, Deramond H, Belkoff SM, eds. Percutaneous Vertebroplasty. New York: Springer-Verlag, 2002:175–180

10. Jensen ME, Evans AJ, Mathis JM, Kallmes DF, Cloft HJ, Dion JE. Percutaneous polymethylmethacrylate vertebroplasty in the treatment of osteoporotic vertebral compression fractures: technical aspects. AJNR Am J Neuroradiol 1997;18:1897–1904

11. Belkoff SM, Mahoney M, Fenton DC, Mathis JM. An in vitro biomechanical evaluation of bone cements used in percutaneous vertebroplasty. Bone 1999;25:23s–26s

12. Belkoff SM, Mathis JM, Erbe EM, Fenton DC. Biomechanical evaluation of a new bone cement for use in vertebroplasty. Spine 2000;25:1061–1064

13. Tohmeh AG, Mathis JM, Fenton DC, Levine AM, Belkoff SM. Biomechanical efficacy of unipedicular versus bipedicular vertebroplasty for the management of osteoporotic compression fractures. Spine 1999;24:1772–1776

14. Belkoff SM, Mathis JM, Jasper LE, Deramond H. The biomechanics of vertebroplasty: the effect of cement volume on mechanical behavior. Spine 2001;26:1537–1541

15. Belkoff SM, Mathis JM, Fenton DC, Scribner RM, Reiley ME, Talmadge K. An ex vivo biomechanical evaluation of an inflatable bone tamp used in the treatment of compression fractures. Spine 2001;26:151–156

16. Belkoff SM, Mathis JM, Deramond H, Jasper LE. An ex vivo biomechanical evaluation of a hydroxyapatite cement for use with kyphoplasty. AJNR Am J Neuroradiol 2001;22:1212–1216

17. Wilson DR, Myers ER, Mathis JM, et al. Effect of augmentation on the mechanics of vertebral wedge fractures. Spine 2000;25: 158–165

18. Jasper LE, Deramond H, Mathis JM, Belkoff SM. The effect of monomer-to-powder ratio on the material properties of Cranioplastic. Bone 1999;25:27s–29s

19. Jasper LE, Deramond H, Mathis JM, Belkoff SM. Material properties of various cements for the use with vertebroplasty. J Mater Sci Mater Med 2002;13:1–5

20. Belkoff SM, Mathis JM, Jasper LE, Deramond H. An ex vivo biomechanical evaluation of a hydroxyapatite cement for use with vertebroplasty. Spine 2001;26:1542–1546

21. Wong W, Mathis JM. Commentary: is intraosseous venography a significant safety measure in the performance of vertebroplasty. J Vasc Interv Radiol 2002;13:137–138

22. Galibert P, Dermond H, Rosat P. [Preliminary note on the treatment of vertebral angioma by percutaneous acrylic vertebroplasty.] (In French) Neurochirurgie 1987;33:166–168

23. Bascoulergue Y, Duquesnel J, Leclercq R. Percutaneous injection of methyl methacrylate in the vertebral body for the treatment of various diseases: percutaneous vertebroplasty [abstract]. Radiology 1988;169:372

24. Cotton A, Dewatre F, Cortet B. Percutaneous vertebroplasty for osteolytic metastases and myeloma. Radiology 1996;200:525–530

25. Weill A, Chiras J, Simon JM. Spinal metastases: indications for and results of percutaneous injection of acrylic surgical cement. Radiology 1996;199:241–247

26. Cyteval C, Sarrabere MP, Roux JO, Thomas E, Jorgensen C, Blotman F. Acute osteoporotic vertebral collapse: open study on percutaneous injection of acrylic surgical cement in 20 patients. AJR Am J Roentgenol 1999;173:1685–1690

27. Barr JD, Barr MS, Lemley TJ, McCann RM. Percutaneous vertebroplasty for pain relief and spinal stabilization. Spine 2000;25: 923–928

28. Zoarski GH, Snow P, Olan WJ, et al. Percutaneous vertebroplasty for osteoporotic compression fractures: quantitative prospective evaluation of long-term outcomes. J Vasc Interv Radiol 2002;13: 139–148

29. Lieberman IH, Dudeney S, Reinhardt MK, Bell G. Initial outcome and efficacy of "kyphoplasty" in the treatment of painful osteoporotic vertebral compression fractures. Spine 2001; 26:1631–1638

30. Olan WJ. Kyphoplasty: Balloon-Assisted Vertebroplasty. ASNR Spine Symposium. Vancouver, BC, May 11–12, 2002:115–117.

31. Agris JM, Zoarski GH, Stallmeyer MJB, Ortiz O. Intravertebral pressure during vertebroplasty: a study comparing multiple delivery systems. Presented at the annual meeting of the American Society of Spine Radiology, Scottsdale, Az. Feb 19–23, 2003.

32. Belkoff.

33. Nussbaum DA, Gailloud P, Murphy K. A review of complications associated with vertebroplasty and kyphoplasty as reported to the food and drug administration medical device related web site. J Vasc Interv Radiol 2004;15:1185–1192

34. Hiwatashi A, Moritani T, Numaguchi Y. Increase in vertebral body height after vertebroplasty. Am J Neuroradiol 2003;24:185–189

35. McKiernan F, Jensen R, Faciszewski T. The dynamic mobility of vertebral compression fractures. J Bone Miner Res 2003;18:24–29

36. Teng MH, Wei CJ, Vei LC et al. Kyphosis correction and height restoration effects of percutaneous vertebroplasty. Am J Neuroradiol 2003;24:1893–1900

37. Mathis JM. Percutaneous vertebroplasty: complication avoidance and technique optimization. Am J Neuroradiol 2003;24:1697–1706

13

Intraoperative Vertebroplasty for Augmentation of Pedicle Screw Instrumentation in Osteoporotic Bone

J. S. SARZIER, D. M. MELTON, AND D. W. CAHILL

Objectives: On completion of this chapter, the reader should be able to describe the indications and technique used for intraoperative vertebroplasty for augmentation of screw purchase and vertebral body strength.

Accreditation: The American Association of Neurological Surgeons is accredited by the Accreditation Council for Continuing Medical Education to sponsor continuing medical education for physicians.

Credit: The American Association of Neurological Surgeons designates this continuing medical education activity for a maximum of 15 credits in Category I of the Physician's Recognition Award of the American Medical Association.

The Home Study Examination is online at www.aans.org/education/books/vertebro.asp

---

Since they were first used by Roy-Camille almost 40 years ago, pedicle screws have gained universal acceptance among spine surgeons.[1–3] They are now used in virtually all posteriorly instrumented lumbar and thoracolumbar procedures and are more recently being used in more cephalad thoracic applications.[4] Pedicle screws are commonly used for the posterior reconstruction of degenerative, traumatic, developmental, oncologic, and infectious spinal lesions. Such screws often allow shorter segment fixation in the lumbar spine and provide several advantages over hook- or wire-fixated constructs in both lumbar and thoracolumbar applications.[5,6] These include more rigid fixation, the ability to manipulate all three columns in instrumented segments, and greater resistance to torsional and flexural failure after surgery. Pedicle-fixated screws are more resistant to failure than pedicle-or lamina-fixated hooks in all testing modes except pullout.[6–10]

In osteoporotic bone, however, pedicle screw pullout is a significant risk. Construct failure secondary to end screw pullout is not uncommon among osteoporotic patients undergoing surgery for various spinal conditions.[11–14] Corollary to the tenuous screw purchase inherent in osteopenic bone is the limitation implied in any manipulative effort applied to effect deformity

correction in such patients. Screws may extrude or fracture the vertebrae into which they are inserted when enough force is applied across them to correct the deformity at hand[15–27] (Fig. 13–1).

In our south Florida practice, hundreds of patients are seen with degenerative deformities superimposed on moderate to severe osteoporosis. Although most of these patients are postmenopausal women, very elderly men and others on chronic steroid or antimetabolite therapy are also commonly seen. Severe osteoporosis is also common among patients with metastatic tumors (often after irradiation) and among those with chronic renal failure–associated osteodystrophy. Sagittal (kyphosis, olisthesis), coronal, or rotational (scoliosis) deformities may be seen. Posterior pedicle screw–fixated constructs applied to such patients have an unacceptably high failure rate if significant corrective force is applied to screw-fixated rods either intra- or postoperatively.

It is our current practice to perform intraoperative transpedicular methylmethacrylate vertebroplasties in vertebrae to be instrumented with pedicle screws immediately before screw placement in such patients in an effort to decrease the risk of screw pullout or fracture with subsequent construct failure.[1]

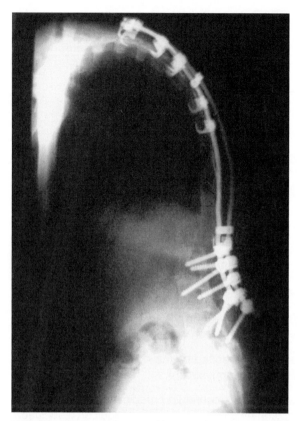

FIGURE 13–1 A 32-year-old severely osteoporotic woman with neurogenic kyphoscoliosis. An attempted correction with a long posterior construct has failed secondary to screw extrusion at the caudal end of the construct with secondary hook dislodgment at the cephalad end. The risk of pedicle screw pullout increases directly with increasing construct length and increasing degree of deformity correction.

■ Preoperative Evaluation

Published data have documented the correlation between decreased bone mineral density and increased risk of pedicle screw pullout in vitro and in vivo.[15,18–20,24,25,27] However, bone densitometry measurements vary greatly with both technique and statistical algorithm.[28–30] Currently, we do not use T-scores to assess the potential need for intraoperative vertebroplasty. Rather, we use a combination of historical, radiographic, and biomechanical assessments always available for any patient, including age and length of time from the menopause; presence or absence of spontaneous compression fractures; smoking history; history of steroid use or radiotherapy to the area to be instrumented; use of estrogen replacement, biphosphonate drugs, or calcitonin; relative obesity; and most importantly, the biomechanical requirements to correct the deformity at hand. Constructs that must correct high-grade kyphotic, scoliotic, or olisthetic deformities, longer constructs, and posterior stand-alone constructs are more likely to fail.

In any patient who does not present with a new or progressive cord-related deficit, every effort is made to ameliorate as many preoperative risk factors as is feasible. Chronic corticosteroid use is minimized or eliminated, if clinically possible. Smoking is discontinued in every case. The use of replacement estrogen, biphosphonate drug, or calcitonin therapy is instituted in every case in which it is clinically safe to do so, though the short-term benefits of any of these treatments are probably negligible. Weight loss is encouraged though rarely with any measurable effect.

The majority of patients among whom intraoperative vertebroplasty is recommended preoperatively have a Jekei grade of three or four on preoperative lateral lumber spine radiographs. Most have spontaneous compression fractures in the thoracic or lumbar spine, most have high-grade kyphoscoliotic deformities, and some have failed a previous attempt at pedicle-fixated fusion. As we have reported elsewhere, in vitro data suggest that intraoperative vertebroplasty of pedicle-instrumented vertebrae redistributes corrective pullout forces from the interface of the screw and pedicle alone to the entire augmented vertebral corpus and its surrounding cortex.[15] In the laboratory, this technique decreases the risk of screw pullout and increases the forces that may be applied to the augmented vertebra without fracture.[26,31–34] We discuss the clinical results using this technique below.

■ Methods and Materials

The growing popularity of percutaneous vertebroplasty and kyphoplasty has resulted in the development of cement delivery devices that are significantly improved over earlier techniques using small bone biopsy needles and small-volume hand injection.[35–41] The newer devices use large-bore bone trocars and threaded piston injection devices with extension tubing sufficiently long as to allow the operator to stand clear of the fluoroscopy beam.[42] At least two companies manufacture and market devices that are equally useful for vertebroplasty injection. Each has subtle advantages and disadvantages that may influence individual operator performance.

Unfortunately, neither system is packaged with the polymer to be injected or with the mandatory barium to make the polymer radiographically visible because neither material is yet approved for this specific indication. Methylmethacrylate designed and packaged specifically for use in vertebroplasty is currently pending before the Food and Drug Administration (FDA). At the moment, only a single company manufactures sterile barium powder suitable for mixing with cranioplasty-type methylmethacrylate powder before adding the liquid catalyst. It should be noted that standard radiographic barium that is often used for gastroenteric studies is unsterile and unsuited in consistency for mixture with methylmethacrylate powder.[43]

There are two other technical innovations that have been widely reported and that may or may not have a place in preinstrumentation vertebroplasty. The first is cannulated and fenestrated pedicle screws.[44] Injection of the polymer directly through such a screw could, in theory, simplify the procedure by eliminating the need for trocar placement with injection before screw placement. At least two issues must be addressed before this technique becomes widely applicable, however. First, the distribution of cement being injected through several fenestrations makes it difficult to control. Injection resistance pressures may be high at the most appropriate screw depth, and manipulation of depth of injection may be difficult if the screw must be repeatedly manipulated. Second, fenestrated screws are inherently weaker and more prone to fracture than solid screws. Both in vitro and in vivo biomechanical testing of any such screw must be accomplished to establish adequate strength and fracture resistance long before market release.

The second technique that may or may not have a role in preinstrumentation vertebroplasty is balloon kyphoplasty. Some have suggested that the larger volume of methylmethacrylate that may be injected after kyphoplasty balloon expansion may improve the strength of the overall construct and further decrease screw pullout resistance. We do not currently employ this technique for several reasons. The most common reason for avoiding this technique is that the vertebrae to be instrumented are usually not fractured or kyphotic. More importantly, the destruction of the boney trabeculae within the vertebral body may weaken the screw interface with the body deep to the pedicle and distribute all such forces to the cortical rim of the vertebra. Balloon kyphoplasty increases the risk of cortical margin fracture that may render subsequent vertebroplasty unsafe for fear of extravasation. We currently believe that simple vertebroplasty using bone trocars and screw/piston injections is the simplest, safest, and most effective technique prior to instrumentation.

The most important technical factor for the performance of intraoperative vertebroplasty is the quality of the fluoroscopy available in the surgical suite. Extravasation and epidural migration of the polymer are often subtle and difficult to visualize without excellent multiplanar imaging. The risks of paravertebral vein extension with subsequent pulmonary embolism or of epidural extension with root or cord compression are too high if inadequate intraoperative visualization cannot be avoided. Both death and paraplegia have been reported following vertebroplasty.[45–51]

Portable C-arm imaging devices suitable for use in the operating suite have been greatly improved in recent years but are still far inferior to the digital, high-intensity devices now in use in fixed (immobile) applications in radiography suites. Safe intraoperative vertebroplasty requires a current-generation digital C-arm image intensifier and a well-trained technician experienced in its use. We still prefer to use a single machine in multiple planes rather than to combine two machines at right angles to one another, which we have found to be too cumbersome and not effective as a time saver.

■ Procedure

A standard posterior subperiosteal exposure is performed to expose the laminae, facets, and transverse processes of all levels to be instrumented. In most cases, anterior and posterior releases are performed via complete Gill laminectomy and posterior interbody diskectomy at all apical and adjacent segments of either coronal or sagittal deformities. This allows complete visualization of the dural tube and exiting nerve roots through their foramina. If necessary, ventral and lateral osteophyte fracture is accomplished via interbody distraction to complete circumferential releases.[52,53] If end-plate integrity is adequate, rectangular posterior lumbar interbody fusion (PLIF) cages packed with autologous bone are placed. If end plates are compromised secondary to osteoporotic fracture, only bone is placed without cages. In most cases, all interbody manipulation is completed before vertebroplasty.

The instrumentation is begun by placement of bilateral trocars through the pedicles of all levels in which preinstrumentation vertebroplasty is planned. This is done using biplanar fluoroscopy. If pedicle size allows, both rostral and caudal end vertebrae are always included along with as many interval segments as is thought practical for a given case. The number of levels in which vertebroplasty is planned depends on the length of the total construct, the severity of the deformity to be corrected (if any), and whether the construct crosses a junctional region of the spine. In most cases, at least two rostral and two caudal levels are planned.

During trocar placement, it is very important to avoid violation of the ventral cortex of the vertebra to prevent extrusion of the cement into the ventral soft tissues. This can usually be assured by placing the tip of the trocar no deeper than the midpoint of the vertebral body as seen on lateral imaging. The inner stylet of the trocar is initially left in place to avoid both bleeding and potential air embolism.

Once trocar positioning is satisfactory, the cranioplasty cement powder (Codman, Raynham, MA) is added to a graduated cylinder containing the chosen aliquot of sterile barium powder (Parallax, Scotts Valley, CA). The amount of barium may be varied according to the imaging requirements in any given patient; 5 cc is usually adequate.

The amount of cranioplasty powder and monomer may also be varied to alter both viscosity and time to polymerization (working time). A thinner mixture (12 cc cranioplasty powder, 7 cc monomer) flows more easily in moderately osteoporotic bone and allows a longer working time but carries a higher risk of venous embolism or extravasation through small fracture lines. A thicker mixture (9 cc powder, 5 cc monomer) is suggested in severely osteoporotic bone. This requires a higher injection pressure and shortens the time to polymerization but is less likely to extravasate through microfractures or to embolize.

After the cranioplast is added to the barium powder, the vial is shaken to disperse the barium within the methylmethacrylate powder. Failure to do this prior to adding the liquid monomer results in the heavier barium remaining at the bottom of the injection vial, and there will be no visualization of the injected cement during lateral fluoroscopy, thus carrying a high risk of pulmonary embolism upon injection.

After the two powders are mixed, the liquid monomer is injected into the cylinder using a sterile syringe and 18-gauge spinal needle. The spinal needle allows for the monomer to be injected in equal amounts into the bottom, middle, and top of the powder mixture. This allows for quicker and more uniform reaction between the liquid and powder. After all of the monomer has been injected, the cylinder is recapped and again shaken to allow further reaction between the liquid and powder as well as keeping the heavy barium from settling as the mixture becomes the consistency of a flowing paste. This is achieved in approximately 2 minutes. The mixture is then poured into the delivery device, being careful to avoid air pockets that may interfere with the controlled injection of the cement. The delivery device is then purged on the back table to allow for filling of the extension tubing. As the cement is purged it should be noted that the first few turns deliver a semi-dry, gritty aliquot followed by the pasty consistency described before. Failure to purge this initial plug of cement can cause obstruction of the trocar or poor control of the cement injection.

The stylet is then removed from one trocar to allow irrigation with saline. The extension tubing is attached to the hub of the trocar and the delivery device is turned at a moderate rate until the barium particles are seen within the confines of the trocar on lateral fluoroscopy. When the particles reach the end of the trocar, it is recommended that the turning of the delivery device be stopped or reversed until the particles are seen to be static on lateral fluoroscopy. At this point it is recommended that the delivery device be turned at increments of one-quarter turn to avoid overpressurizing the system. After each quarter turn is completed, the

particles will be noted to continue to flow secondary to the compliance within the tubing. The next turn may be started when the flow is noted to slow or stop. This injection technique ensures that if the cement begins to fill unwanted areas, then the pressure may be released or reversed with less than a half turn of the delivery device. Injection must be done under continuous fluoroscopic visualization. If the fluoroscopy is interrupted, the delivery device must be turned in reverse one full turn to avoid continued flow due to residual pressure within the system.[42]

As the cement is injected, the margins are noted to have a nebulous appearance. It is important to evaluate the flow in two planes *several* times during the injection. One must be vigilant to observe for circumscribed or round-appearing cement collections appearing in the midline of the body in either the posteroanterior (PA) or lateral views because this may be early filling of paravertebral or epidural veins. More eccentric circumscribed collections may represent filling of fractures that may extend into the disk space or paravertebral soft tissues. If abnormal collections are noted, there are a few options to keep from further injection into the unwanted spaces. The first is to simply stop injection for 1 to 2 minutes. The cement within the body sets up faster than that in the injection device secondary to the difference between the room and body temperatures. After waiting a period of time, resume injection very slowly and observe for expansion of the undesired collection. If the above technique is unsuccessful, one may withdraw the needle approximately one quarter of its depth and resume slow injection. The cement will likely follow a path of least resistance through the weakened bone and not advance into the thickening cement. The trocar should be slowly withdrawn and cement injected to allow placement of cement back toward the pedicle, but injection directly at the base or into the pedicle is unnecessary and dangerous even when a Gill laminectomy is performed and extravasated cement may be directly visualized and removed. A third option is to disconnect the delivery device from the first trocar and begin injecting the contralateral trocar. This again allows the cement already injected to set up while proceeding with the procedure.

The amount of cement to inject into each side is variable and dependent on the degree of successful filling and the presence of unwanted collections. When an interbody fusion has been performed, it is important to avoid complete end-plate to end-plate body filling to preserve viable end-plate bone (Fig. **13–2**). The average volume is between 2 and 4 cc of cement and the working time is from 8 to 12 minutes.

After injection of the cement, the delivery device is disconnected from the trocar and the trocar is removed. Failure to do so results in formation of a vacuum that pulls cement into the pedicle. The pedicle should not

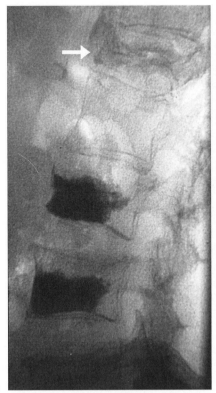

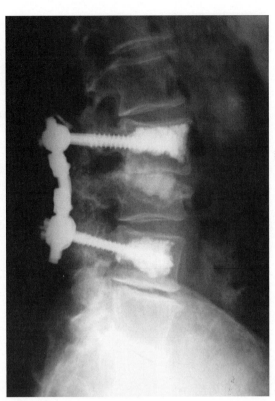

A   **B**

FIGURE 13–2 (A) Intraoperative vertebroplasties performed in preparation for instrumented correction of fracture seen at arrow. A caudal screw trajectory is planned and no interbody fusion between vertebroplastied segments is planned. **(B)** Correction of the failed stand-alone posterior lumbar interbody fusion (PLIF) procedure referred after fracture of vertebrae caudal to PLIF grafts. Polymethylmethacrylate (PMMA) cement is placed away from the end plates of the vertebrae in which interbody fusion is planned.

be tapped because the cement will foul the tap. The screws are placed in the usual fashion otherwise and to the same depth as the trocar. To aid screw placement, a system with a self-tapping flute is recommended. Attention is then turned to the next level and the procedure is repeated. At completion of placement of all augmented screws, it is recommended that the cement be allowed to completely harden prior to attempting to compress or distract. Saving a small sample from the last delivery device allows one to judge when manipulation of the construct is safe. When the last sample becomes exothermic and fully hardened, then all the augmented levels have fully cured and manipulation may proceed.

■ Results

We have now employed intraoperative preinstrumentation vertebroplasty in more than 30 osteoporotic patients and more than 100 vertebral levels. In vitro studies in our laboratories suggested that vertebroplasty augmentation does not return screw pullout resistance to "normal" levels but does shift the point of failure from the pedicle to the cortical wall of the vertebral body. This increased the pullout resistance of Jekei grade 4 severely osteoporotic vertebrae to a resistance comparable to nonaugmented Jekei grade 1 or 2 vertebrae.[15]

Clinical experience has verified this laboratory result. In all nine levels in which there have been fixation failures of pedicle screws in vertebroplastied vertebrae, the failure has been by fracture of the vertebral body with the vertebroplastied portion of the body remaining attached to the implanted screw. There have been no screw pullouts (Fig. **13–3**).

To this point, we have had no infections in vertebroplastied vertebrae. Although we have seen several instances in which early filling of paravertebral veins with methylmethacrylate is documented (Fig. **13–3**), we have had no cases of pulmonary embolism. We have had no cases of epidural or foraminal extravasation with cord or root compression.

There have been eight cases in which intraoperative vertebroplasty has allowed us to salvage previously failed procedures (Fig. **13–4**). It is our subjective impression that the deformity corrections obtained while employing preinstrumentation vertebroplasty are more anatomically complete than would have been otherwise possible (Figs. **13–5** and **13–6**).

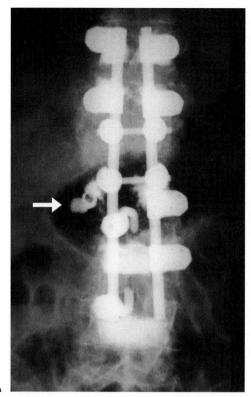

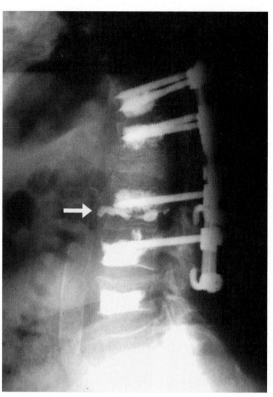

A

B

FIGURE 13–3 Anteroposterior (AP) and lateral radiographs of the four-level instrumented correction of kyphotic deformity secondary to osteoporotic compression fracture. Extravasation of methylmethacrylate into paravertebral veins is seen at the arrows. Hooks have been used to salvage the left side of the caudal fixation point after fracture of the vertebral body during corrective manipulation.

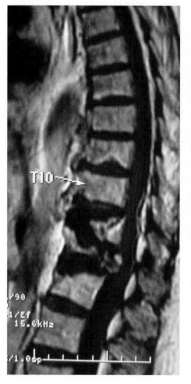

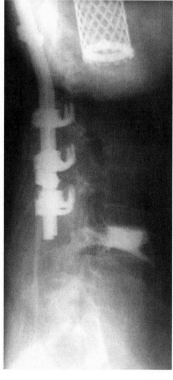

A

B

FIGURE 13–4 (A) A 36-year-old rheumatoid after many years of steroid therapy. Lateral T1-weighted magnetic resonance imaging (MRI) reveals lytic destruction of T11, T12, and part of L1. Patient was paraparetic. **(B)** Initial 360-degree reconstruction using cage anteriorly and clawed-hook fixated rods posteriorly. Three sets of down-going hooks cephalad to the cage (not seen in this view) and three sets of upgoing sublaminar hooks caudal to the cage were used.

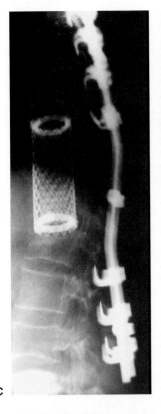

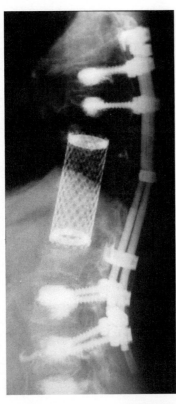

C   **D**

FIGURE 13–4 (*Continued*) **(C)** Three days after surgery, when the patient was mobilized, the two most caudal laminae fractured with secondary construct failure. **(D)** Repair using preinstrumentation vertebroplasty and pedicle screws two levels cephalad and two levels caudal to anterior device. Downgoing sublaminar hooks supplement the rostralmost screws.

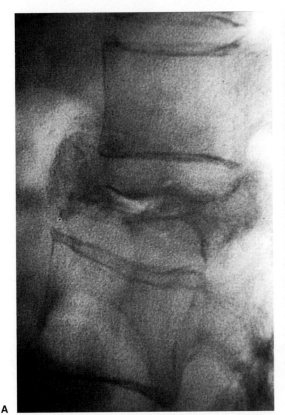

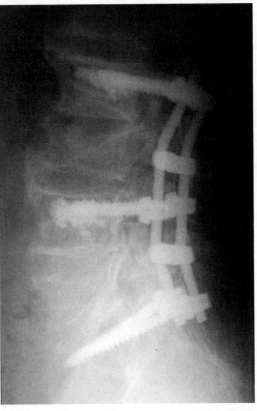

A   **B**

FIGURE 13–5 (A) Osteoporotic compression fracture with vertebra plana at L3. Lesser compression fracture with 20% height loss at L5 is not visualized in this film. **(B)** Reconstruction using intraoperative vertebroplasties of L2 and L4 instrumented segments and bicortical screws in S1 allows gratifying restoration of height at both L3 and L5. Distractive force necessary to obtain reduction would likely have resulted in construct failure in the absence of vertebroplasties.

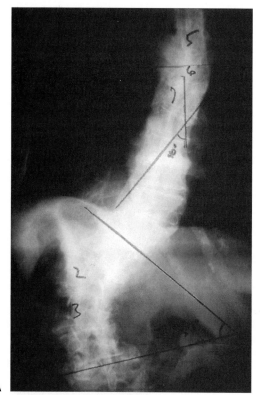

A

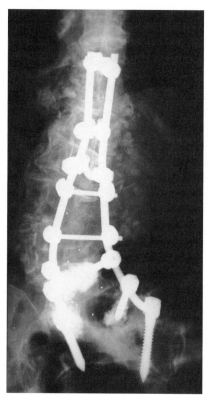

B

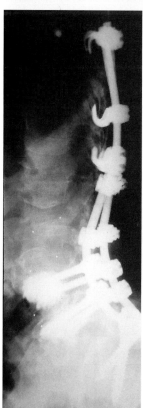

C

FIGURE 13–6 (A) Octogenarian with marked osteoporosis and severe postlaminectomy scoliosis. **(B,C)** Correction using intraoperative vertebroplasties at the caudal end of the construct and hooks at the cephalad end allow rebalancing in the coronal plane and adequate restoration of lordosis. In the absence of vertebroplasties, caudal end screw extrusion would have been a significant risk.

The greatest drawbacks to the procedure are the additional 15 to 20 minutes per level required in the operating room (OR) to accomplish it and the greatly increased x-ray exposure to OR personnel. Experience tends to decrease both these risks.

■ Discussion

It must be remembered that the current bipedicular vertebroplasty technique usually leaves a relatively empty, unaugmented area between the two halves of the treated vertebra. Significant corrective forces applied to the vertebroplasty-fixated screw leads to failure at this weak point. Vertebroplasty augmentation does *not* return severely osteoporotic vertebrae to the normal state. Although corrective forces that may be successfully applied are increased when compared with unaugmented osteoporotic vertebrae, they are still measurably less than might be safely applied to young, nonosteoporotic vertebrae. The likelihood of instrumented vertebral failure is directly proportional to the force applied to it. The risk of failure is decreased by increasing the number of anterior and posterior releases performed, increasing the number of augmented vertebrae to be instrumented, and by supplementing screw-fixated levels with same-level hooks.[11-13]

Spine surgery performed in osteoporotic patients still has a significant risk of failure. Intraoperative vertebroplasty of vertebrae to be instrumented with pedicle screws is a valuable technique that does appear to decrease the risk of construct failure by pedicle screw extrusion.[54] As such, we recommend it in selected cases. Excellent fluoroscopic visualization in at least two planes and careful, slow injection technique are mandatory if potentially disastrous complications are to be avoided. Failure by fracture of augmented vertebral bodies may still occur. Careful pre- and postoperative attention to the elimination of risk factors and to the therapy of the underlying osteoporosis is critical. A fundamental understanding of the biomechanical requirements of the case at hand dictate the design of any restorative construct. Vertebroplasty augmentation of vertebrae to be instrumented should always be applied first to those vertebrae at greatest risk of failure by screw extrusion. In most cases, these are the vertebrae at the ends of any long construct, vertebrae on the fixed side of the junctional zones, and vertebrae at the apical portions of coronal deformities.

REFERENCES

1. Roy-Camille R, Saillant G, Mazel C. Internal fixation of the lumbar spine with pedicle screw plating. Clin Orthop 1986;203:7–17
2. Roy-Camille R, Saillant G, Berteaux D, Salgado V. Osteosynthesis of thoraco-lumbar spine fractures with metal plates screwed through the vertebral pedicles. Reconstr Surg Traumatol 1976;15:2–16
3. Roy-Camille R, Roy-Camille M, Demeulenaere C. Osteosynthesis of dorsal, lumbar, and lumbosacral spine with metallic plates screwed into vertebral pedicles and articular apophyses. Presse Med 1970;78:1447–1448
4. Heller JG, Shuster JK, Hutton WC. Pedicle and transverse process screws of the upper thoracic spine: biomechanical comparison of loads to failure. Spine 1999;24:654–658
5. Yuan HA, Garfin SR, Dickman CA, Mardjetko SM. A historical cohort study of pedicle screw fixation in thoracic, lumbar, and sacral spinal fusions. Spine 1994;19(20 Suppl):2279S–2296S
6. Hirabayashi S, Kumano K, Kuroki T. Cotrel-Dubousset pedicle screw system for various spinal disorders: merits and problems. Spine 1991;16:1298–1304
7. Hackenberg L, Link T, Liljenqvist U. Axial and tangential fixation strength of pedicle screws versus hooks in the thoracic spine in relation to bone mineral density. Spine 2002;27:937–942
8. Gayet LE, Pries P, Hamcha H, Clarac JP, Texereau J. Biomechanical study and digital modeling of traction resistance in posterior thoracic implants. Spine 2002;27:707–714
9. Myers BS, Belmont PJ Jr, Richardson WJ, Yu JR, Harper KD, Nightingale RW. The role of imaging and in situ biomechanical testing in assessing pedicle screw pull-out strength. Spine 1996;21:1962–1968
10. Liljenqvist U, Hackenberg L, Link T, Halm H. Pullout strength of pedicle screws versus pedicle and laminar hooks in the thoracic spine. Acta Orthop Belg 2001;67:157–163
11. Hasegawa K, Takahashi HE, Uchiyama S, et al. An experimental study of a combination method using a pedicle screw and laminar hook for the osteoporotic spine. Spine 1997;22:958–962
12. Chiba M, McLain RF, Yerby SA, Moseley TA, Smith TS, Benson DR. Short-segment pedicle instrumentation: biomechanical analysis of supplemental hook fixation. Spine 1996;21:288–294
13. Suzuki T, Abe E, Okuyama K, Sato K. Improving the pullout strength of pedicle screws by screw coupling. J Spinal Disord 2001;14:399–403
14. Coe JD, Warden KE, Herzig MA, McAfee PC. Influence of bone mineral density on the fixation of thoracolumbar implants: a comparative study of transpedicular screws, laminar hooks, and spinous process wires. Spine 1990;15:902–907
15. Sarzier JS, Evans AJ, Cahill DW. Increased pedicle screw pullout strength with vertebroplasty augmentation in osteoporotic spines. J Neurosurg Spine 2002;96:309–312
16. Brantley AG, Mayfield JK, Koeneman JB, Clark KR. The effects of pedicle screw fit: an in vitro study. Spine 1994;19:1752–1758
17. Polly DW Jr, Orchowski JR, Ellenbogen RG. Revision pedicle screws: bigger, longer shims–what is best? Spine 1998;23:1374–1379
18. von Strempel A, Kuhle J, Plitz W. Stability of pedicle screws, II: Maximum pullout force with reference to bone density. Z Orthop Ihre Grenzgeb 1994;132:82–86
19. Halvorson TL, Kelley LA, Thomas KA, Whitecloud TS III, Cook SD. Effects of bone mineral density on pedicle screw fixation. Spine 1994;19:2415–2420
20. Soshi S, Shiba R, Kondo H, Murota K. An experimental study on transpedicular screw fixation in relation to osteoporosis of the lumbar spine. Spine 1991;16:1335–1341
21. Hirano T, Hasegawa K, Takahashi HE, et al. Structural characteristics of the pedicle and its role in screw stability. Spine 1997;22:2504–2509
22. Hirano T, Hasegawa K, Washio T, Hara T, Takahashi H. Fracture risk during pedicle screw insertion in osteoporotic spine. J Spinal Disord 1998;11:493–497
23. McLain RF, Fry MF, Moseley TA, Sharkey NA. Lumbar pedicle screw salvage: pullout testing of three different pedicle screw designs. J Spinal Disord 1995;8:62–68
24. Bennett GJ, Serhan HA, Sorini PM, Willis BH. An experimental study of lumbar destabilization: restabilization and bone density. Spine 1997;22:1448–1453

25. Hadjipavlou AG, Nicodemus CL, al-Hamdan FA, Simmons JW, Pope MH. Correlation of bone equivalent mineral density to pull-out resistance of triangulated pedicle screw construct. J Spinal Disord 1997;10:12–19

26. Wittenberg RH, Lee KS, Shea M, White AA III, Hayes WC. Effect of screw diameter, insertion technique, and bone cement augmentation of pedicular screw fixation strength. Clin Orthop 1993;296: 278–287

27. Okuyama K, Sato K, Abe E, Inaba H, Shimada Y, Murai H. Stability of transpedicle screwing for the osteoporotic spine: an in vitro study of the mechanical stability. Spine 1993;18:2240–2245

28. El-Hajj Fuleihan G, Stock JL, McClung MR, Saifi G. A national random survey of bone mineral density reporting in the United States. J Clin Densitom 2002;5:3–9

29. Bolotin HH. Analytic and quantitative exposition of patient-specific systematic inaccuracies inherent in planar DXA-derived in vivo BMD measurements. Med Phys 1998;25:139–151

30. Valkema R, Verheij LF, Blokland JA, et al. Limited precision of lumbar spine dual-photon absorptiometry by variations in the soft-tissue background. J Nucl Med 1990;31:1774–1781

31. Cameron HU, Jacob R, Macnab I, Pilliar RM. Use of polymethyl-methacrylate to enhance screw fixation in bone. J Bone Joint Surg Am 1975;57:655–656

32. Flahiff CM, Gober GA, Nicholas RW. Pullout strength of fixation screws from polymethylmethacrylate bone cement. Biomaterials 1995;16:533–536

33. Motzkin NE, Chao EY, An KN, Wikenheiser MA, Lewallen DG. Pull-out strength of screws from polymethylmethacrylate cement. J Bone Joint Surg Br 1994;76:320–323

34. Yerby SA, Toh E, McLain RF. Revision of failed pedicle screws using hydroxyapatite cement: a biomechanical analysis. Spine 1998;23:1657–1661

35. Hardouin P, Fayada P, Leclet H, Chopin D. Kyphoplasty. Joint Bone Spine 2002;69:256–261

36. Amar AP, Larsen DW, Esnaashari N, Albuquerque FC, Lavine SD, Teitelbaum GP. Percutaneous transpedicular polymethylmethacrylate vertebroplasty for the treatment of spinal compression fractures. Neurosurgery 2001;49:1105–1114

37. Garfin SR, Yuan HA, Reiley MA. New technologies in spine: kypho-plasty and vertebroplasty for the treatment of painful osteoporotic compression fractures. Spine 2001;26:1511–1515

38. Belkoff SM, Mathis JM, Fenton DC, Scribner RM, Reiley ME, Talmadge K. An ex vivo biomechanical evaluation of an inflatable bone tamp used in the treatment of compression fracture. Spine 2001;26:151–156

39. Heini PF, Walchli B, Berlemann U. Percutaneous transpedicular vertebroplasty with PMMA: operative technique and early results:

a prospective study for the treatment of osteoporotic compression fractures. Eur Spine J 2000;9:445–450

40. Bostrom MP, Lane JM. Future directions: augmentation of osteoporotic vertebral bodies. Spine 1997;22(24 suppl):38S–42S

41. Jensen ME, Evans AJ, Mathis JM, Kallmes DF, Cloft HJ, Dion JE. Percutaneous polymethylmethacrylate vertebroplasty in the treatment of osteoporotic vertebral body compression fractures: technical aspects. AJNR Am J Neuroradiol 1997;18:1897–1904

42. Al-Assir I, Perez-Higueras A, Florensa J, Munoz A, Cuesta E. Percutaneous vertebroplasty: a special syringe for cement injection. AJNR Am J Neuroradiol 2000;21:159–161

43. Leibold RA, Gilula LA. Sterilization of barium for vertebroplasty: an effective, reliable, and inexpensive method to sterilize powders for surgical procedures. AJR Am J Roentgenol 2002;179:198–200

44. McKoy BE, An YH. An injectable cementing screw for fixation in osteoporotic bone. J Biomed Mater Res 2000;53:216–220

45. Scroop R, Eskridge J, Britz GW. Paradoxical cerebral arterial embolization of cement during intraoperative vertebroplasty: case report. AJNR Am J Neuroradiol 2002;23:868–870

46. Kaufmann TJ, Jensen ME, Ford G, Gill LL, Marx WF, Kallmes DF. Cardiovascular effects of polymethylmethacrylate use in percutaneous vertebroplasty. AJNR Am J Neuroradiol 2002;23:601–604

47. Aebli N, Krebs J, Davis G, Walton M, Williams MJ, Theis JC. Fat embolism and acute hypotension during vertebroplasty: an experimental study in sheep. Spine 2002;27:460–466

48. Ryu KS, Park CK, Kim MC, Kang JK. Dose-dependent epidural leakage of polymethylmethacrylate after percutaneous vertebroplasty in patients with osteoporotic vertebral compression fractures. J Neurosurg Spine 2002;96:56–61

49. Harrington KD. Major neurological complications following percutaneous vertebroplasty with polymethylmethacrylate: a case report. J Bone Joint Surg Am 2001;83-A:1070–1073

50. Ratliff J, Nguyen T, Heiss J. Root and spinal cord compression from methylmethacrylate vertebroplasty. Spine 2001;26:E300–E302

51. Padovani B, Kasriel O, Brunner P, Peretti-Viton P. Pulmonary embolism caused by acrylic cement: a rare complication of percutaneous vertebroplasty. AJNR Am J Neuroradiol 1999;20:375–377

52. Brantigan JW, Steffee AD. A carbon fiber implant to aid interbody lumbar fusion: two-year clinical results in the first 26 patients. Spine 1993;18:2106–2107

53. Brantigan JW, Steffee AD, Geiger JM. A carbon fiber implant to aid interbody lumbar fusion: mechanical testing. Spine 1991; 16(6 suppl):S277–S282

54. Wuisman PI, Van Dijk M, Staal H, Van Royen BJ. Augmentation of (pedicle) screws with calcium apatite cement in patients with severe progressive osteoporotic spinal deformities: an innovative technique. Eur Spine J 2000;9:528–533

14

Vertebroplasty in Private Practice: Training, Credentialing, Billing, and Marketing

JEFFREY D. GROSS

Objectives: On completion of reading this chapter, the spine surgeon should be able to understand and describe how to establish a program for vertebroplasty in the setting of a private practice.

Accreditation: The American Association of Neurological Surgeons is accredited by the Accreditation Council for Continuing Medical Education to sponsor continuing medical education for physicians.

Credit: The American Association of Neurological Surgeons designates this continuing medical education activity for a maximum of 15 credits in Category I of the Physician's Recognition Award of the American Medical Association.

The Home Study Examination is online at www.aans.org/education/books/vertebro.asp

Neurosurgeons and orthopedic spine surgeons who have separated from their academic heritage must continue to be prepared to offer their patients the latest and most minimally invasive treatment techniques when appropriate. Community-based private practices often serve a well-informed patient base and must be able to provide a level of care often at the cutting edge, and above the standard of care because it will be demanded. It is not uncommon to encounter sophisticated patients who present to the office with information from the media, including the Internet, and with questions regarding procedures that may be at a level beyond a surgeon's recent experience, such as minimally invasive treatment. Patients want appropriate surgical treatment with the least pain, smallest incision, and shortest "down time" away from their occupations and daily activities. Thus it is imperative to stay abreast of recent developments in neurosurgical treatments and techniques. With that underlying theme, this chapter discusses implementing a vertebroplasty program in private practice.

Historically, painful osteoporotic compression fractures have been treated with bed rest and analgesics. Healing is often slow and can be largely incomplete. New applications of standard medical acrylics through minimally invasive approaches have led to the popularity of the surgical treatment of these fractures: vertebroplasty and

kyphoplasty. These minimally invasive surgical techniques are particularly suited for the elderly, who most commonly manifest such fractures. Additionally, their surgical candidacy for larger reconstructive procedures is poor. Such treatment can offer new life to patients who used to be crippled by such fractures and their complications. For the purposes of this chapter, the term *vertebroplasty* is used to encompass all of the available techniques and variations of the minimally invasive surgical treatment of painful osteoporotic compression fractures covered elsewhere in this book, including kyphoplasty.

Establishment of a program to provide vertebroplastic treatment to the patient community of a spine surgeon's private practice involves appropriate technique training, instruction of the operating room staff, receipt of appropriate credentials, and acquisition of knowledge for successful marketing and billing practices. This chapter provides information concerning these topics, based on the experience of a vertebroplasty program in the private practice setting.

■ Training

Appropriate surgical technique training for the performance of any new procedure may be satisfied in many ways:

through residency training, through courses, or through directly observing a surgeon already knowledgeable and skilled in the desired techniques, followed by practice in a nonclinical setting (i.e., cadaver laboratory). Vertebroplasty is only just now being taught in the residency setting. However, some orthopedic and neurosurgical residents and fellows still have minimal exposure to these techniques. Furthermore, community hospital medical credentialing officers may not be familiar with such techniques, and because of the need for support from both the radiology department as well as the operating room, reluctance may be encountered.

Perhaps the most straightforward way to train to perform a vertebroplasty is by attending a specific course on the topic. Such courses are often given by national medical organizations during meetings. Other methods of satisfying training requirements are through courses for surgeons that are sponsored by companies. One company requires training with its equipment on cadaveric specimens before being allowed to utilize their technique (Kyphon, Santa Clara, CA). Surgeons who satisfactorily complete the requirements of these 1- or 2-day courses are given a certificate, which is helpful for obtaining hospital credentials to perform vertebroplasties.

Another way to obtain surgical training in vertebroplastic techniques is to spend time watching an expert, such as a surgeon who has significant experience in performing such procedures. Choosing such a mentor can be as simple as calling the author of a paper or poster on vertebroplasty. Alternatively, one could network through neurosurgical, orthopedic, or other medical organizations to find out who in a certain region is offering such a procedure. A request to observe someone, particularly someone out of one's primary field, should be personal and should present no threat of competition for patients. An interested surgeon may consider traveling for a day or two to watch several procedures. If this method of training is chosen, nonclinical practice on cadaver or animal specimens should be included to gain experience handling the tools and getting a "feel" for cannulating a pedicle from the small skin incision.

The above-mentioned approaches to training should not be considered replacements for the expected basic anatomic knowledge of the region, the need for review of the available literature concerning the techniques, and a critical appraisal of the utility of the technique in a given patient population. Learning through the mistakes of others can help ensure success for such technique-dependent procedures. Furthermore, one should not embark on performing such procedures unless a certain comfort level has been satisfied. This can only be measured by the trainee and should not be clouded by ego or machismo. Vertebroplasties, although minimally invasive, have real and potentially lethal complications. These potential morbidities can be easily manifested

in elderly patients who have a high incidence of severe pulmonary, cardiac, and endocrinologic disease without much physiologic "reserve."

■ Credentialing

Ultimately, surgeons seeking to begin a vertebroplasty program must satisfy not only their own comfort level with the knowledge and training for this new procedure but also that of the local medical staff and/or facility. Most hospitals and surgery centers have credentialing rules for existing and new procedures. Often, this process involves a period of proctoring by an experienced surgeon once the training is complete. In some settings, documentation of training is adequate to allow the performance of vertebroplasties. However, in this age of seemingly unlimited liability, most hospital staffs stipulate proctorship by either a physician who has performed the procedure or another physician observer who can at least attest that the procedure was performed with appropriate skill.

If the requirement is to provide a proctor who is a surgeon well versed in vertebroplasty, one must often recruit such an expert from an academic center or facility where vertebroplasties are performed. This person may not always practice the same specialty but should have a modicum of experience with the procedure before agreeing to proctor someone seeking credentials. Accommodating arrangements should be made to avoid disrupting the proctor's schedule. Perhaps multiple procedures could be scheduled sequentially when more than one is required by the medical staff. Often, visiting proctors do not have medical privileges at the facility where proctoring is required, but these can often be granted on a temporary basis for this purpose. Discussions regarding liability surrounding those temporary privileges should be made with the medical staff office and the proctor because many professional liability policies cover only procedures performed at the proctor's usual hospitals. The proctor should be given the opportunity to be a co-surgeon or assistant surgeon, and should be thanked with a gift for his/her time.

In facilities that allow another surgeon without vertebroplasty experience to proctor, one should be careful to choose someone who either will be a partner or will not be competing for vertebroplasty patients in the same market. Some community markets may be quite competitive in the spinal surgery arena. Thus a surgeon should likely not choose a surgeon from a competing group unless a particular surgeon is stipulated by the medical staff, and no other suitable alternatives exist. It may be wiser to import an expert from far away, even if one has to defray the travel costs, so as not to be incurring competition.

There is no formal accreditation credential for a facility doing vertebroplasty. Although credentialing of the operating room staff is not required, appropriate training should be made available. This training may be provided by companies that market and sell products and kits for the performance of vertebroplasties. The staff should practice mixing and handling the acrylic as well as the delivery devices to best assist the surgeon during the procedure. It cannot be overemphasized how important it is to familiarize the fluoroscopy technicians with the necessary views required to perform a vertebroplasty. It is often necessary to rotate a single fluoroscope back and forth between the anteroposterior (AP), lateral, and pedicle (owl's eyes) views, each of which requires particular finesse to achieve adequate alignment given a kyphotic deformity, rotated position, degenerative scoliosis, or other radiologic obstacles.

It is helpful to inform in writing the medical staff and surgery committees before beginning a vertebroplasty program; describe the procedure, the staff and equipment needs, and the dedication needed to bringing this service to the hospital. This written information will also help develop interest in the program and garner support for its success from the hospital administration and medical staff. It may even lead to referrals.

■ Reimbursement

Reimbursement for vertebroplasties is almost always based on Medicare rates because the overwhelming majority of patients with painful osteoporotic compression fractures are over the age of 65. Exceptions will be younger patients with secondary osteoporosis, or those with pathologic fractures; however, the current procedural terminology (CPT) coding will be the same. The reader is cautioned that regulations regarding the use of CPT codes for various procedures and the identity of these codes are not static and change over time. The description of billing practices below represents the author's experience at the present time and should not serve as a substitute for published CPT guidelines.

Billing for vertebroplasties should be the same for any other open procedure. Despite the fact that the incisions to allow placement of the trocars are small, the procedure is still an "open" one and is subject to the same workup, surgical decision making, intraoperative care, and postoperative management as any other open spine surgery. In fact, one may argue that performing minimally invasive open surgery requires additional training, skill, and experience beyond that of standard open surgery and should be rewarded financially on at least an equal basis. Thus, to document the procedure as it was performed, the operation report should specify the incision made for the placement of a trocar or needle.

The operative report should describe the facet block if local anesthetic is used (even if the patient is placed under general anesthesia). If antibiotics are used in the acrylic, this should be described. However, there is no perfect code for this part of the procedure. Utilization of CPT code 62310 (thoracic) or 62311 (lumbar) probably best describes the intraosseous antibiotic injection than do codes 90782 to 90799.

Injection of contrast material to identify the vertebral venous system is a venogram and may be billed as such. The injection of acrylic into the vertebral body represents an intravertebral body arthrodesis with polymethylmethacrylate (PMMA). If a kyphotic reduction is made (kyphoplasty), then it should be so stated in the operative report and may be billed as a deformity reduction. The modifier–79 may be utilized for this code and for the intrabody arthrodesis code if the patient returns with a new vertebral compression fracture within the 90-day postoperative period. The new vertebroplasty codes 22520 (thoracic), 22521 (lumbar), and 22522 (additional level) now replace the 22851 (thoracic) or 22852 (lumbar) intravertebral body device/arthrodesis code but reimburse at a much lower rate.

Additionally, one may perform a bone biopsy if there is suspicion of pathologic disease in the fracture before the placement of acrylic material. Bilateral modifiers can be used if the vertebroplasty was performed from both sides. There are also new codes for the supervision and interpretation of intraoperative fluoroscopic images.

Controversial reimbursement issues concerning the procedures have been debated. Some insurance carriers and regional Medicare agencies have not reimbursed appropriately for the procedures as they have been performed, due to their minimally invasive nature. These payers believe that the small incision to allow trocar placement does not adequately represent the level of surgical service provided to these patients, and they might not reimburse for the open fracture reduction code, and sometimes not for the intrabody arthrodesis code. Some surgeons have utilized the unlisted spine code (22899) but have had difficulty receiving reimbursement for vertebroplasties coded in this way. Payers are often reluctant to reimburse for miscellaneous CPT codes. For the purposes of efficiency of reimbursement, this code is not suggested. Medicare began reimbursing for an unlisted spinal procedure code (22899) in some regions, which effectively lowered the reimbursement as compared with a traditional open spinal fracture reduction.[1] A separate code for kyphoplastic reduction (above and beyond vertebroplasty) may be developed to reduce reimbursement even further. These new vertebroplasty and kyphoplasty codes should be considered experimental by billers and payers. It is unclear at this time which services and other codes the nationally accepted reimbursement policies will ultimately encompass (and therefore disallow payment as part of a vertebroplasty).

TABLE 14–1 Typical Procedures That May Be Billed for Vertebroplasty, Depending on the Level of Service and Assuming a Single Level

Procedure 2001	CPT Code*
Facet block, (bilateral modifier–51)	64470
Bone biopsy, (bilateral modifier–51)	20225
Venogram, (bilateral–51)	36005
Open reduction of deformity, (bilateral–51)	22327 (t), 22325 (l)
Open reduction, additional level (bilateral–51)	22328
Intrabody arthrodesis with PMMA, (bilateral–51)	22851(t), 22852 (l)
Injection of antibiotic, (bilateral–51)	62310 (t), 62311 (l)
Supervision and interpretation of fluoroscopy	76012 (per level)

t, thoracic; l, lumbar.

*Actual reimbursement for these codes depends on the payer, region, and documentation. CPT codes shown are from the 2003 Current Procedural Terminology Handbook.[2] [Note: there are relatively new vertebroplasty codes 22520 (thoracic), 22521 (lumbar), and 22522 (additional level), which may be used to replace the intravertebral body device code if appropriate].

These new codes do not, in the author's opinion, represent the level of service provided for this procedure.

Table 14–1 lists the procedures that typically may be billed for a vertebroplasty, depending on how the procedure was performed. An overnight stay is usually required by the facility for Medicare reimbursement, although these procedures can often be performed on an outpatient basis.

Surgeons should be actively involved in driving the Health Care Financing Administration (HCFA) and other payer organizations, as well as elected politicians to preserve appropriate reimbursement for vertebroplasties. If reduced, the reimbursement will not reflect the level of training, time, and effort of patient workup and postoperative management, the skill level required to perform the procedure and enable the identification and management of potential complications (even requiring additional surgery), the assumption of professional liability, and the additional skill and training required to implement minimally invasive techniques such as these. In Pennsylvania, the complete cessation of reimbursement for vertebroplasties occurred following two perioperative deaths. Although appropriate investigation of these cases is required, it is imprudent of payers to make unilateral medical decisions. Preventing the effective treatment of the ongoing and crippling pain from untreated osteoporotic vertebral fractures should not be the purview of insurance companies and government agencies. Thus active letter writing and other communications with CEOs

of HMOs and with politicians should help deliver the message regarding the utility and necessary reimbursement of vertebroplasties. Physicians who perform these procedures are likewise obligated to report their results so as to demonstrate the efficacy of these procedures.

■ Successful Marketing

Since few orthopedic or neurological surgeons have the time or inclination to obtain an MBA, this information about marketing is presented to help provide ideas to jump-start referrals for patients needing vertebroplasties. The best way to reach one's local medical community is to offer a continuing medical education (CME) class or grand-rounds lecture. This is an excellent way to inform the local referring physicians about the availability of vertebroplasties in their community. Many primary care physicians are not exposed to the latest developments in spinal surgery and may not even have heard of this procedure. It is helpful to have an instructive slide show and brochures, some of which are provided by the companies that market equipment for vertebroplasties.

An excellent way to reach the local emergency department staff is to make a brief presentation at their periodic meetings. The staff will enjoy this nonadministrative agenda item, and the presentation may lead to the referral of patients who present acutely. It is a good idea to offer to do consults for these patients, even when you are not on call, particularly if no one else in the community offers vertebroplasties.

A simple mailing containing copies of one or two useful journal articles or brochures and a business card is a good way to reach geriatricians, endocrinologists, rheumatologists, and primary care physicians. Offer to visit the offices of larger practices to give a lunchtime presentation. This is a nice way to develop referral patterns for other aspects of spinal surgical care as well. Also, physical therapy centers enjoy having visiting surgeons discuss procedures, particularly of the spine.

Ultimately, any efforts to let patients and referring physicians know that your vertebroplasty services are available will open avenues of consultations for patients to benefit from your new program.

REFERENCES

1. National Hertage Insurance Company Final Local Medical Review Policy. September 2001:53–59
2. American Medical Association. Current Procedural Terminology 2001. Chicago: AMA Press, 2001

15

Emerging Techniques and Technologies for Percutaneous Vertebral Augmentation

ROHAM MOFTAKAR, BRIAN P. WITWER, AND DANIEL K. RESNICK

Objectives: On completion of this chapter, the reader should be able to discuss emerging technologies for use in vertebroplasty and kyphoplasty.

Accreditation: The American Association of Neurological Surgeons is accredited by the Accreditation Council for Continuing Medical Education to sponsor continuing medical education for physicians.

Credit: The American Association of Neurological Surgeons designates this continuing medical education activity for a maximum of 15 credits in Category I of the Physician's Recognition Award of the American Medical Association.

The Home Study Examination is online at www.aans.org/education/books/vertebro.asp

Percutaneous vertebroplasty (PVP) was developed by Galibert et al in 1984 for the treatment of hemangiomas involving the spine.[1] This method was later extended to treat osteoporotic compression fractures, osteolytic metastasis, and myeloma of the spine.[2] PVP affords immediate mechanical stabilization and also offers patients rapid pain relief.[3] This procedure is now becoming more popular for the treatment of vertebral compression fractures. During vertebroplasty a 10- to 15-gauge cannula is passed through the pedicle under image guidance, followed by injection of cement into the cancellous interior of the vertebral body.[1] The main goal of PVP is to maximize cement deposition within the vertebral body while minimizing damage to the adjacent tissue. Because this technique is fairly new, there are new technologies constantly emerging designed to improve the safety, ease, and outcome of this procedure.

This chapter presents an overview of some recently developed products and techniques used in vertebroplasty. These new devices and cements are intended to improve safety, improve ease of application, and improve outcome. The reader should be cautioned that many of these devices are not specifically approved by the Food and Drug Administration (FDA) for use in vertebroplasty.

■ Bone Substitutes for Vertebroplasty: Polymethylmethacrylate (PMMA) and Newer Cements

An ideal augmentation material for vertebroplasty must have several important properties. First, the bone substitute must be easy to apply in terms of ease of handling, the mixing procedure, and the percutaneous application of the material through cannulas. The material must have low initial viscosity, but not so low that it easily extravasates. Radiopacity is also important so that the cement flow can be followed with intraoperative fluoroscopy. The setting time of the material should be predictable and reasonable, and the viscosity of the cement should remain constant during the period of application. The heat given off should be minimal. The material should provide immediate reinforcement of the vertebral body and allow early ambulation of the patient. Stiffness and yield strength should be similar to natural bone. The augmentation should be long lasting. The material must not cause adverse reactions to the surrounding tissue. Finally, the bone substitute must be cost-effective.

Polymethylmethacrylate (PMMA) is currently the most commonly used bone cement. Long-term studies have shown that PMMA is highly durable and secondary fractures are very rare.[4] The PMMA cements most commonly used are Simplex P (Stryker-Howmedica-Osteonics, Rutherford, NJ), Cranioplastic (DePuy International Ltd., Blackpool, England), and Palacos LV 40.[5] PMMA is relatively inexpensive and cures to a solid in ~5 minutes. Handling characteristics and the setting time can be altered by changing the mixture of monomer to solvent. A recent study of the relative strength and stiffness of vertebral bodies (VBs) augmented with various commercially available cements suggests that augmentation with Simplex P results in vertebral body stiffness restoration and significant increase in strength.[6] However, it should be noted that to improve cement visualization under fluoroscopy, agents such as barium sulfate must be added and may have an effect on the curing time and ultimate strength.

The use of PMMA in PVP is associated with several potential complications: (1) the high polymerization temperature may lead to surrounding tissue damage; (2) differences in the mechanical strength of injected and noninjected adjacent VB may lead to secondary fractures; and (3) leakage of PMMA into adjacent anatomic structures may cause neural, vascular, or pulmonary insult.[7]

In an effort to improve the safety and efficacy of vertebroplasty and kyphoplasty, newer bone cements as well as osteoconductive materials in a granular form have been developed. Among these osteoconductive granular materials are hydroxyapatite, a mixture of bovine type I collagen and hydroxyapatite/tricalcium phosphate, and plaster of paris. Coral has also been used in Europe for percutaneous vertebroplasty with good success (Fig. 15–1). Its radiodensity is different from that of bone, allowing good radiographic follow-up evaluation of its resorption. Cunin et al[7] evaluated the use of coral from the point of injectability, biocompatibility, and osteoconductivity. They found that injection of coral granules into osteoporotic thoracic vertebral bodies of cadavers was easy to achieve and led to a homogeneous filling of the vertebral bodies. They injected coral at various concentrations within vertebral bodies to attain good interlocking between coral granules and bone trabeculae. This group also injected coral into sheep vertebral bodies by using invasive surgical methods. There was no coral granule migration into adjacent structures or venous system during the surgical procedure. In addition, bones filled with coral granules demonstrated increased osteogenesis in comparison with the cavities left empty, confirming the osteoconductivity of coral. The effect of coral granule injection on pain relief remains to be determined. Similarly, the biomechanical effects of coral injection are not defined.

Bisphenol-a-glycidyl dimethacrylate (bis-GMA) resins, which have been used in orthopedic applications for

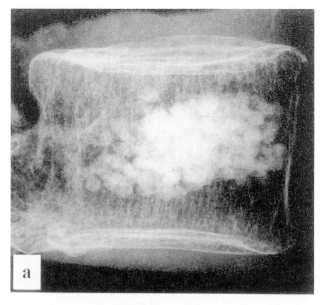

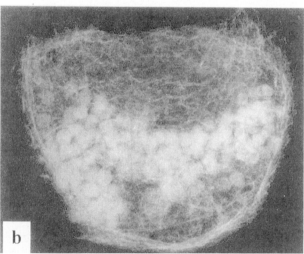

FIGURE 15–1 X-ray demonstrating an osteoporotic human cadaver vertebral body (**A**, lateral; **B**, apical) injected with coral granules. (From Cunin et al[7] with permission.)

more than 20 years, are another class of cements that might be of a potential use in vertebroplasty. Various formulations of bis-GMA have been developed to reduce the amount of monomers spilled from the site of deposition, to reduce high local temperature, and to enhance direct bone contact. One such formula is Cortoss (Orthovita, Malvern, PA) synthetic cortical bone void filler, a biocompatible, bone bonding, terpolymer cortical bone substitute containing bis-GMA, bisphenol-a-ethoxy dimethacrylate (bis-EMA), and triethylene glycol dimethacrylate (TEGDMA) resins reinforced with synthetic glass-ceramic particles to stimulate bone apposition at the interface, barium boroaluminosilicate glass for radiopacity and strength, and silica for improved viscosity (Fig. 15–2). Erbe et al[4] compared the biocompatibility

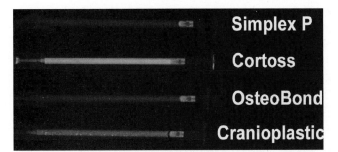

FIGURE 15–2 Comparison of radiopacity of Cortoss to other cements such as Simplex P, OsteoBond, and Cranioplastic. (From Orthovita CD Rom Presentation, Orthovita, Malvern, PA 19355, with permission.)

and interfacial bond strengths of Cortoss with a commercially available PMMA, Simplex P, by implanting these two materials in rabbit femurs for up to 52 weeks and in sheep long bones for up to 78 weeks. This group reported that new periosteal and endosteal bone was formed within defects sites filled with either Cortoss or Simplex P, but the initial response was greater with Cortoss than with Simplex P. Furthermore, the periphery of Cortoss implants were invaded by new blood vessels, which supported the hypothesis of osteogenesis. This group concluded that Simplex P was generally unreactive in terms of bone formation. In addition, although both Cortoss and Simplex P were surrounded by bone at 52 weeks in sheep and 24 weeks in rabbits, half of the Simplex P specimens were separated from bone by a layer of fibrous connective tissue at 24 weeks. In terms of ability to bond to bone, displacement forces were greater for rods held in place with Cortoss than with Simplex P at every time point examined throughout the 78 weeks of the study. The authors attributed the greater stability of the bone/Cortoss interface to a faster initial bone response and a greater degree of mineralization around Cortoss.

Another similar bioactive cement, Orthocomp (Orthovita, Malvern, PA), has been developed that may also overcome some of the deficiencies of PMMA mentioned above. Orthocomp is a bioactive, glass-ceramic–reinforced composite material with a matrix of Bis-GMA, Bis-EMA, and TEGDMA. One of the features of Orthocomp that distinguishes it from PMMA is its lower exotherm property.[1] This material is naturally more radiopaque than PMMA cements with even 20% barium sulfate content, which should be advantageous when it is used to detect inadvertent extravasation. Orthocomp is not resorbable, but the hydrophilic surface allows bone to bond chemically to the cement. Belkoff et al[1] studied the effect of Orthocomp on stabilizing osteoporotic compression fractures and how its performance compares with that of Simplex P. This study was done on osteoporotic cadaveric vertebral bodies. The results of this study demonstrated

that osteoporotic vertebral bodies treated with either Orthocomp or Simplex P were significantly stronger than they were in their initial conditions. However, vertebral bodies augmented with Orthocomp were significantly stronger than vertebral bodies augmented with Simplex P. Augmentation with Orthocomp resulted in restoration of initial stiffness, whereas augmentation with Simplex P did not restore initial vertebral body stiffness. This suggests that smaller volumes of Orthocomp may be adequate for augmentation of osteoporotic vertebral fractures. The questions that still have to be addressed regarding Orthocomp are the effect of fill volume on the mechanical properties of repaired osteoporotic compression fractures, the risk of cement extravasation and embolization, the potential reduction of micromotion at the fracture site, and the effects of vertebroplasty with this cement on pain associated with vertebral compression fractures.

BoneSource (Stryker-Howmedica-Osteonics, Rutherford, NJ), a hydroxyapatite cement, which is currently approved by the FDA as a cranial defect filler, has been proposed for use in vertebroplasty. The absence of exothermic property and the known osteoconductivity of hydroxyapatite may suggest that it is a better choice than PMMA cements. However, the difficulty with introducing this material into the vertebral body due to poor flow characteristics has made this material difficult to use. Belkoff et al[6] compared the biomechanical effectiveness of BoneSource prepared with methylcellulose to Simplex P containing 10% $BaSO_4$ standard formulation and Simplex P with additional $BaSO_4$ (30%). This study was done on cadaveric thoracic and lumber vertebral bodies. This group's data suggested that BoneSource restored initial vertebral body strength, but it did not augment vertebral body strength to the level achieved by Simplex P. In addition, BoneSource, similar to the two preparations of Simplex P, did not fully restore stiffness. Belkoff et al also reported that the use of methylcellulose solution to mix BoneSource provided a cement that was easily injected to vertebral body using 11-gauge cannulas, although slightly more effort was required for injection as compared with the Simplex P formulations. However, difficulties in injection were experienced when BoneSource was mixed with sterile water, as recommended in the product insert. It is currently unclear how BoneSource may respond in vivo in a weight-bearing condition, because this material is used currently as cranial defect filler in a non–weight-bearing environment. In addition, there is no information regarding the utility of hydroxyapatite for pain relief following vertebroplasty.

Schildhauer et al[8] reported on the in vitro use of a carbonated apatite cement (Norian, Cupertino, CA) in augmentation of vertebral bodies. Norian's action in situ is nonexothermic and forms an osteoconductive carbonated apatite that is similar chemically to the mineral phase of bone. In their study looking at 10 lower thoracic vertebral bodies, this group concluded that injection of Norian provided increased energy absorption beyond 25% collapse of the vertebrae under compressive loading, suggesting that injection of this apatite cement would be mechanically effective for patients with significant osteoporotic spines. They also concluded that injection of Norian could be performed in a minimally invasive fashion. The fact that this cement is osteoconductive would mean that it can support the trabecular structure initially and should be replaced by new bone formation over time.

Kurashina et al[9] have developed a new calcium phosphate cement consisting of α-tricalcium phosphate (α-TCP), dicalcium phosphate dibasic (DCPD), and tetracalcium phosphate monoxide (TeCP) (Biopex, Central Research Institute, Mitsubishi Materials, Yokoze, Chichibu, Japan). This group has shown in a previous study that this cement has good biocompatibility and can form a direct union with bone tissue. In their current study they evaluated tissue response to this cement by using it in a rabbit mandibular model. They report that there were no adverse effects observed in the surrounding tissue (according to histologic studies). This group also reported that there was direct contact between cement and bone without intervention of soft tissue. However, in four of 16 specimens, the cement paste implant was lost shortly after implantation. The authors emphasize that in those cases intense bleeding occurred after creating a defect in the mandible and continuous bleeding after implantation eliminated the cement. Several authors, including Munting et al, have emphasized hemostasis as an important criteria for setting of cements. Kurashina et al[9] also report that Biopex cement is resorbable in tissue by dissolution and digestion by phagocytic cells.

Another calcium phosphate bone substitute is (ABS) (α-BSM, ETEX Corp., Cambridge, MA). Knaack et al[10] studied this bone substitute in a rabbit and canine model and reported that this material is similar to the mineral component of bone and demonstrated nearly complete resorption within 1 to 2 months following implantation. After implantation new bone was observed to form concomitant with resorption of the cement. They also report that this material is endothermic when hardening initiates. Because the cement requires heat to activate the hardening process, the hydrated paste remains workable for several hours at room temperature. Bai et al[11] demonstrated that α-BSM compares favorably with PMMA for strengthening vertebral bodies in cadaveric spines. With α-BSM the fracture strength was significantly stronger than in the intact group. Stiffness was also significantly higher than control groups. α-BSM was able to partially restore anterior height of the vertebral bodies (60%).

Another calcium phosphate–based bone cement is Biocement H. This is a powder consisting of α-tertiary

calcium phosphate and some precipitated hydroxyapatite. Khairoun et al[12] found that aqueous solutions resembling blood had no effect on its setting behavior. They also report that this material has good osteointegration in matter of days followed by osteotransduction within months. No further information is available regarding mechanical properties of Biocement H.

■ New Technologies to Decrease Complications in Vertebroplasty

Galibert and Deramond introduced PVP with PMMA as an augmentation procedure in 1987.[13] PMMA is the most commonly used bone cement for PVP in the United States[14]; however, several disadvantages have been described.[5] PMMA leakage out of the vertebral body into paravertebral tissue has been reported in as many as 60% of patients.[15] In addition, PMMA gives off a strongly exothermic reaction with excess heat generated during in situ polymerization up to 110°C.[16] This temperature is sufficient to induce bone and tissue necrosis. Although leakage of PMMA producing cord compression or radiculopathy is rare, it has been reported.[15] There have been multiple reports of adverse cardiovascular events such as pulmonary embolism, severe arterial hypotension, bradycardia, bronchospasm, and asystole in the use of PMMA in hip arthroplasty. There has been one case report of injection of PMMA during vertebroplasty resulting in transient arterial hypotension.[14,34]

Schildhauer et al[8] have described a suction-injection technique that the authors report has many advantages. First, they report that the pressure applied to the cement specimens significantly increased the ultimate compression strength of the cement and eliminated differences measured without pressure. The pressure presumably reduced the amount of air trapped within the fluid cement during setting. Injection alone as used to introduce PMMA in clinical practice could result in high intravertebral pressures. This would force cement into the low-pressure system of the spine venous plexus, causing pulmonary embolism and perhaps neurologic deficits. The authors claim that the suction-injection technique should reduce the chance of such problems. In addition, washing the site of the cement injection with suction allows better infiltration of the cement than injection alone, and the cement can be introduced with minimal pressure. In this study the suction-injection technique was effective in vitro such that half of the cadaveric thoracic vertebral bodies were infiltrated with cement. The limitation of this method in the study is that it has not been tried in vivo.

Verlaan et al[17] have reported their experience with balloon vertebroplasty for direct restoration and augmentation of the anterior column after distraction and

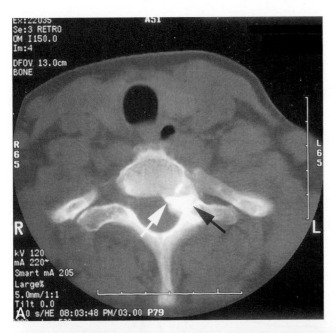

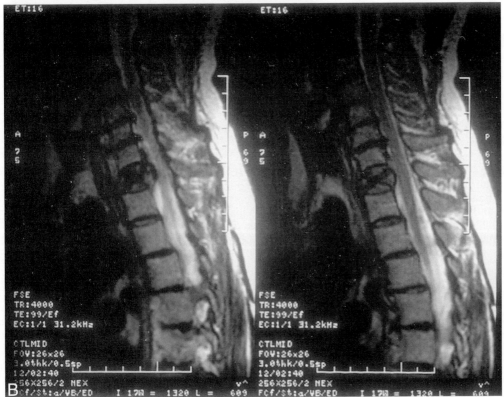

FIGURE 15–3 (A) An axial computed tomography (CT) demonstrating compromise of T1 foramina and spinal canal by methylmethacrylate (arrows). **(B)** T2-weighted sagittal magnetic resonance imaging (MRI) showing cord compression. (From Ratliff et al,[15] with permission.)

posterior fixation of thoracolumbar vertebral fractures in a human cadaver model (Fig. **15–3**). These authors inserted inflatable bone tamps designed for kyphoplasty procedure (KyphX, Kyphon, Inc., Sunnyvale, CA) into both pedicles of the fractured vertebra and advanced them until the final paramedian localization in the anterior third of the vertebral body. Then, using fluoroscopy, the position of the inflatable bone tamps was checked. The bone tamps were inflated by gradually forcing a radiopaque fluid from a pressure-gauge–equipped syringe

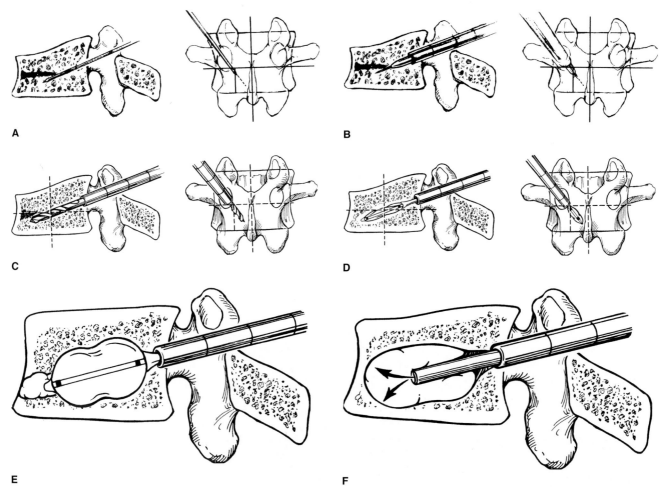

A

B

C

D

E

F

FIGURE 15–4 (A) Drawing of a guide pin entering the pedicle in the lateral (left) and anteroposterior (right) plane. **(B)** A stylet and cannula are placed over the guide pin into the pedicle. **(C)** The guide pin and stylet are removed. This is followed by a hand-driven drill to create a larger channel in the bone. **(D)** The drill is removed and the bone tamp is then inserted. **(E)** The balloon is inflated. This creates a cavity and compacts the bone around the balloon, elevating the fractured cortices. **(F)** The balloon is removed, a bone filler device is inserted through the cannula, and cement is injected (packed) into the void. (From Garfin et al,[19] with permission.)

into the balloons. With every milliliter of added volume the balloons were checked with fluoroscopy. Inflation was continued until reduction of the end plate was achieved. Subsequently both balloons were deflated and retracted after satisfactory reduction. Then BoneSource was injected until a complete filling of the defect was achieved fluoroscopically. The authors favor this method because the inflatable bone tamps facilitate end-plate reduction and by simultaneous creation of a bone void, cement could be injected under low pressure. This decreases the risk of leakage of the cement, which is one of the complications of cement injection under pressures. Clinical studies to evaluate the usefulness of this procedure are currently under way.

Belkoff et al[18] evaluated the use of inflatable bone tamp (tamp) in their cadaveric spine model to see whether the tamp restores vertebral height in simulated compression fractures and whether this results in vertebral body strength and stiffness values different from those obtained using percutaneous vertebroplasty alone (Figs. **15–4** and **15–5**). These authors experienced extravasation of cement with use of PVP but not in vertebroplasty treated with the tamp. Also, use of the tamp resulted in significantly greater height restoration than in PVP. Only vertebral bodies treated with the tamp returned to initial stiffness.

■ Advances in Delivery Systems and Techniques

The goal of vertebroplasty is to maximize cement deposition within the vertebral body while minimizing damage to adjacent tissue. The conventional technique of

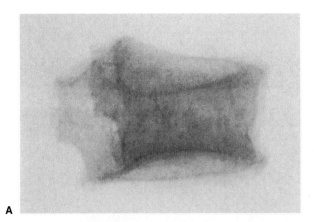

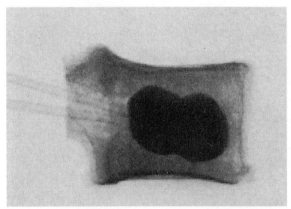

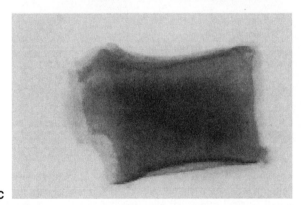

FIGURE 15–5 Lateral x-ray of a vertebral body after initial compression **(A)**, after tamp inflation **(B)**, and after injection of cement **(C)**. (From Belkoff et al,[18] with permission.)

vertebroplasty requires cement filling through bilateral injections.[19] Cannulating the contralateral pedicle places additional neural structures at risk and prolongs the procedure. Also, multilevel fractures requiring multilevel cannulation may be too invasive for procedures performed under local anesthesia. Visualization of cement injection through a second pedicle cannulation is often obscured by the indwelling cement from the first injection, potentially increasing the risk for venous or epidural cement extravasation. A unipedicular approach may simplify and increase the safety of the vertebroplasty procedure.

Tohmeh et al[20] reported the biomechanical efficacy of unipedicular vertebroplasty. Unipedicular cement injections restored osteoporotic cadaveric vertebral body stiffness to intact values. No significant differences were observed in stiffness and strength when comparing unipedicular and bipedicular cement augmentation of vertebral bodies.

Kim et al[21] studied the radiographic and clinical outcomes in a group of patients subjected to unipedicular injection. They noted that filling across the midline was achieved in 96% of injections. Pain relief was similar in both the unipedicular and bipedicular approaches.

The modified unipediculate approach described by Kim et al[21] uses a different fluoroscopic localization technique. The anteroposterior (AP) fluoroscopic tube is angled more laterally until the oval appearance of the pedicle is transformed into the appearance of a Scottish terrier dog. The facet joint is positioned more medially to the eye of the Scottie dog. The central aspect of the oval is entered with the needle. The needle enters the pedicle lateral to the superior articulating facet. The needle is advanced until it approaches the anterolateral wall of the contralateral half of the vertebra. Initial cement deposition occurs in the contralateral half of the vertebral body. The ipsilateral half of the body is filled as the needle is retracted across the vertebral body.[21]

Cannula placement is an important first step in obtaining satisfactory filling patterns with vertebral augmentation materials. As discussed above, unipedicular approaches have achieved effective vertebral body reinforcement equal to bipedicular cannulation.[20] Cement deposition using a monopedicular approach, however, may be hindered by front-opening cannulas, which direct the cement flow anteriorly, toward the periphery of the vertebral body, increasing the risk of cement leakage into adjacent veins. Side-opening cannulas were developed to avoid this problem and improve vertebral body filling through a monopedicular approach.

Heini et al[5] demonstrated that the use of a side-opening cannula improved the cement-filling pattern in monopedicular vertebroplasty. The cadaveric vertebral body was divided into four equal zones. The use of the side-opening catheter allowed filling into zone 3 in six out of eight specimens compared with only three out of eight with the front-opening cannula (Fig. **15–6**). Extravasation of cement was noted only in the specimens filled with a front-opening catheter. The authors concluded that the side-opening catheter improved the cement-filling pattern, redirecting the cement flow toward the center of the vertebral body, preventing extravasation of cement into the vessels.[5]

Vertebroplasty of one vertebral level demands rapid controlled instillation of 5 to 15 mL of PMMA through a disposable biopsy needle. Standard 20- and 10-mL

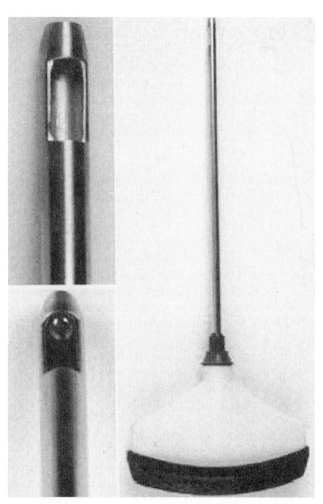

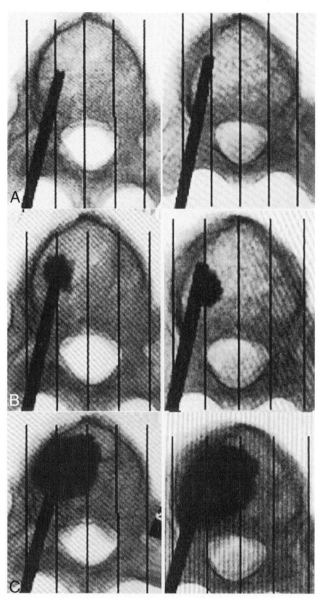

FIGURE 15–6 (Left) Dual-opening cannula. The opening in the end allows for precise insertion of the cannula over a guidewire. This opening then is occluded with a metal ball (lower right). The remaining side opening is used for controlled injection of bone cement directed medially toward the center of the vertebral body (lower right). (Right) Comparison of flow behavior between front-opening (left) and side-opening (right) cannulas. **(A)** The needles are placed identically at the junction of zones 1 and 2. **(B)** After injection of 2 mL, the cement is mainly in area 2 with the side-opening cannula. **(C)** After the full 8 mL is injected, the cement is distributed into zone 3 inches both cases. (From Heini and Dain Allred,[5] with permission.)

push-plunger syringes cannot produce adequate pressure to smoothly inject the volume through the biopsy needle. Flanges of the standard 10-mL syringe deform readily during injection of PMMA, resulting in premature injection failure. Schallen et al[22] developed a flange converter that permits injections of full volumes of a 10-mL syringe as needed, even as injection pressure rises with increasing viscosity during curing (Fig. **15–7**). Of course, the potential for extravasation increases as the pressure used to inject the increases.

■ Additional Uses of Vertebroplasty

Vertebroplasty may augment traditional stabilization techniques in the osteoporotic spine. Spinal fixation relies on the formation of a strong purchase between the hardware and the bone interface with pedicle and vertebral body.[23] Osteoporosis is frequently found in patients undergoing spinal fusion and has been implicated in hardware failure.[24] Augmentation of the screw/bone interface has been attempted by many

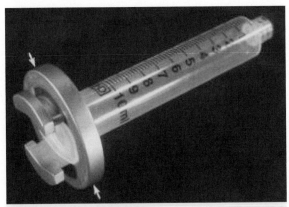

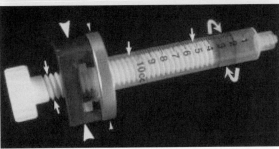

FIGURE 15–7 (Top) Reusable stainless steel flange converter (arrows) with 10-mL standard syringe (optional hub lock not shown). (Bottom) Ten-milliliter syringe has a hard screw-plunger mechanism (straight arrows) that passes through the black plastic hub lock (large arrowheads), which is locked to the flange converter (small arrowheads). The black rubber sealing tip (curved arrows) on the screw interfaces with and pushes the PMMA through the syringe. (From Schallen and Gilula,[22] with permission.)

different techniques including those using composites and PMMA.[24,25] PMMA has been used primarily as a salvage technique after intraoperative pedicle stripping or pedicle fracture. Soshi et al[26] reported insignificant biomechanical advantages in screw pullout strength with augmentation in severe osteoporosis. The use of formal vertebroplasty prior to pedicle screw fixation may provide an adequate screw/bone interface for future pedicle screw fixation. Sarzier et al[27] demonstrated that augmentation of osteoporotic vertebrae in PMMA-assisted vertebroplasty could significantly increase pedicle screw pullout forces to levels exceeding the strength of cortical bone. Biomechanical studies were performed on screws placed in osteoporotic cadaveric thoracolumbar spines augmented with PMMA using a standard verte-broplasty technique. The maximum attainable force appears to be twice the pullout force of the nonaugmented pedicle screw for each osteoporotic grade.

Traumatic fractures of the thoracolumbar junction are occasionally treated by distraction and posterior hardware fixation.[28] Procedural failures after a posterior fixation of a thoracolumbar burst fracture have been reported as high as 45%.[28,29] Posterior fixation failures are felt to be

secondary to the lack of anterior column support. To prevent it, many centers treat these types of fractures with restoration of the anterior column through an anterior surgical approach and strut grafting.[30] Another possible technique for restoration of the anterior column is through vertebral body stabilization using vertebroplasty techniques. Verlaan et al[17] demonstrated in an experimental traumatic fracture model that balloon vertebroplasty with calcium phosphate cement safely restored end-plate integrity of fractures distracted and fixated with short-segment pedicle screws and rods.

■ Image Guidance

The use of frameless stereotactic techniques has revolutionized cranial and spinal procedures. Understanding the complex relationships between the neural, vascular, and bony anatomy is crucial in spinal surgery and stabilization.[31] The use of image guidance permits placement of spinal hardware safely without the use of traditional fluoroscopic and radiographic guidance. In many instances these techniques assist in verifying anatomic relationships of bony anatomy relative to the surrounding neural structures. The basis of these techniques requires fixed verifiable anatomic reference points overlayed onto radiographic anatomic images on fluoroscopy, computed tomography (CT), and magnetic resonance imaging (MRI). This requires internal bony reference points as well as a reference arc anchored to a stationary spinal landmark such as a spinous process or facet.

Vertebroplasty requires precise placement of the cannula within the vertebral body. Similar to the guidance of a pedicle screw into a vertebral body, cannula insertion requires navigating the pedicle body interface without compromising surrounding structures. Currently confirmation of a correct trajectory through a percutaneous approach is performed with continuous fluoroscopic guidance. Three-dimensional navigation is verified with two-dimensional imaging. The exact location of the needle in relationship to the pedicle and its body is estimated by the fluoroscopic image. The use of frameless stereotactic techniques may allow for safer and more accurate needle placement prior to the injection of cement.

Currently, percutaneous techniques do not allow for referencing of stereotactic images to the patient's anatomy. Possible future advancements in external fixation devices providing for anatomic referencing may alleviate this problem. Salehi and Ondra[32] discussed one possible technique for pedicle screw fixation. Using a two-stage technique, fiducial screws were implanted into the posterior elements of the vertebra. A CT scan was obtained, formatted for the frameless stereotactic unit. During the second stage of surgery, registration is performed using the internal fiducial markers. An adaptation

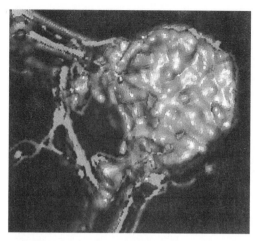

FIGURE 15–8 Three-dimensional CT scan reconstructed image showing the PMMA filling the injected lumbar vertebra. (From Peters et al,[33] with permission.)

of this technique may permit fixation of the reference arc to the patient's bony anatomy prior to obtaining stereotactic images. This may allow for referencing the patient's spinal anatomy to this point of reference. Advances in cranial registration may also be adapted for spinal percutaneous procedures. The creation of laser scanned surface images in relationship to a fixed reference point might allow for laser scanning of the thoracolumbar surface anatomy for stereotactic registration. If registration of the lumbar spine can be performed accurately and reproducibly, frameless stereotaxy might assist in accurate guidance of the vertebroplasty cannula.

Understanding the degree of vertebral augmentation with biosynthetic compounds is crucial in safely reconstructing the pathology of the osteoporotic fracture. The precise location of the vertebral cements is verified using barium-impregnated cement under continuous fluoroscopy. The flow pattern of the cement is continuously observed as it fills the vertebral body. Currently, this process is performed using two-dimensional images. Performing vertebroplasty in a CT-guided suite may permit injection of the contrast-impregnated compound while performing three-dimensional CT scans to identify the volume and location of compound in relationship to surrounding neural and vascular structures. This might allow for instillation of a maximum volume of material while avoiding the extravasation of material into the neural canal or embolization of the venous plexus.

REFERENCES

1. Belkoff SM, Mathis JM, Erbe EM, et al. Biomechanical evaluation of a new bone cement for use in vertebroplasty. Spine 2000; 25:1061–1064

2. Cotten A, Boutry N, Cortet B, et al. Percutaneous vertebroplasty: state of the art. Radiographics 1998;18:311–320

3. O'Brien JP, Sims JT, Evans AJ. Vertebroplasty in patients with severe vertebral compression fractures: a technical report. AJNR Am J Neuroradiol 2000;21:1555–1558

4. Erbe EM, Clineff TD, Gualtieri G. Comparison of a new bisphenol-a-glycidyl dimethacrylate-based cortical bone void filler with polymethyl methacrylate. Eur Spine J 2001;10(suppl 2):S147–S152

5. Heini PF, Dain Allred C. The use of a side-opening injection cannula in vertebroplasty: a technical note. Spine 2002;27:105–109

6. Belkoff SM, Mathis JM, Jasper LE, et al. An ex vivo biomechanical evaluation of a hydroxyapatite cement for use with vertebroplasty. Spine 2001;26:1542–1546

7. Cunin G, Boissonnet H, Petite H, et al. Experimental vertebroplasty using osteoconductive granular material. Spine 2000;25: 1070–1076

8. Schildhauer TA, Bennett AP, Wright TM, et al. Intravertebral body reconstruction with an injectable in situ-setting carbonated apatite: biomechanical evaluation of a minimally invasive technique. J Orthop Res 1999;17:67–72

9. Kurashina K, Kurita H, Hirano M, et al. In vivo study of calcium phosphate cements: implantation of an alpha-tricalcium phosphate/dicalcium phosphate dibasic/tetracalcium phosphate monoxide cement paste. Biomaterials 1997;18:539–543

10. Knaack D, Goad ME, Aiolova M, et al. Resorbable calcium phosphate bone substitute. J Biomed Mater Res 1998;43:399–409

11. Bai B, Jazrawi LM, Kummer FJ, et al. The use of an injectable, biodegradable calcium phosphate bone substitute for the prophylactic augmentation of osteoporotic vertebrae and the management of vertebral compression fractures. Spine 1999;24:1521–1526

12. Khairoun I, Boltong MG, Driessens FC, et al. Effect of calcium carbonate on clinical compliance of apatitic calcium phosphate bone cement. J Biomed Mater Res 1997;38:356–360

13. Heini PF, Berlemann U. Bone substitutes in vertebroplasty. Eur Spine J 2001;10(suppl 2):S205–S213

14. Kaufmann TJ, Jensen ME, Ford G, et al. Cardiovascular effects of polymethylmethacrylate use in percutaneous vertebroplasty. AJNR Am J Neuroradiol 2002;23:601–604

15. Ratliff J, Nguyen T, Heiss J. Root and spinal cord compression from methylmethacrylate vertebroplasty. Spine 2001;26:E300–E302

16. Moreau MF, Chappard D, Lesourd M, et al. Free radicals and side products released during methylmethacrylate polymerization are cytotoxic for osteoblastic cells. J Biomed Mater Res 1998;40:124–131

17. Verlaan JJ, van Helden WH, Oner FC, et al. Balloon vertebroplasty with calcium phosphate cement augmentation for direct restoration of traumatic thoracolumbar vertebral fractures. Spine 2002;27: 543–548

18. Belkoff SM, Mathis JM, Fenton DC, et al. An ex vivo biomechanical evaluation of an inflatable bone tamp used in the treatment of compression fracture. Spine 2001;26:151–156

19. Garfin SR, Yuan HA, Reiley MA. New technologies in spine: kyphoplasty and vertebroplasty for the treatment of painful osteoporotic compression fractures. Spine 2001;26:1511–1515

20. Tohmeh AG, Mathis JM, Fenton DC, et al. Biomechanical efficacy of unipedicular versus bipedicular vertebroplasty for the management of osteoporotic compression fractures. Spine 1999; 24:1772–1776

21. Kim AK, Jensen ME, Dion JE, et al. Unilateral transpedicular percutaneous vertebroplasty: initial experience. Radiology 2002;222: 737–741

22. Schallen EH, Gilula LA. Vertebroplasty: reusable flange converter with hub lock for injection of polymethylmethacrylate with screw-plunger syringe. Radiology 2002;222:851–855

23. Louis R. Fusion of the lumbar and sacral spine by internal fixation with screw plates. Clin Orthop 1986;203:18–33

24. Kostuik JP, Errico TJ, Gleason TF. Techniques of internal fixation for degenerative conditions of the lumbar spine. Clin Orthop 1986;203:219–231

25. Moore DC, Maitra RS, Farjo LA, et al. Restoration of pedicle screw fixation with an in situ setting calcium phosphate cement. Spine 1997;22:1696–1705

26. Soshi S, Shiba R, Kondo H, et al. An experimental study on transpedicular screw fixation in relation to osteoporosis of the lumbar spine. Spine 1991;16:1335–1341

27. Sarzier JS, Evans AJ, Cahill DW. Increased pedicle screw pullout strength with vertebroplasty augmentation in osteoporotic spines. J Neurosurg Spine 2002;96:309–312

28. Parker JW, Lane JR, Karaikovic EE, et al. Successful short-segment instrumentation and fusion for thoracolumbar spine fractures: a consecutive 41/2-year series. Spine 2000;25:1157–1170

29. Kramer DL, Rodgers WB, Mansfield FL. Transpedicular instrumentation and short-segment fusion of thoracolumbar fractures: a prospective study using a single instrumentation system. J Orthop Trauma 1995;9:499–506

30. Kaneda K, Taneichi H, Abumi K, et al. Anterior decompression and stabilization with the Kaneda device for thoracolumbar burst fractures associated with neurological deficits. J Bone Joint Surg Am 1997;79:69–83

31. Truwit CL, Liu H. Prospective stereotaxy: a novel method of trajectory alignment using real-time image guidance. J Magn Reson Imaging 2001;13:452–457

32. Salehi SA, Ondra SL. Use of internal fiducial markers in frameless stereotactic navigational systems during spinal surgery: technical note. Neurosurgery 2000;47:1460–1462

33. Peters KR, Guiot BH, Martin PA, Fessler RG. Vertebroplasty for osteoporotic compression fractures: current practice and evolving techniques. Neurosurgery 2002;51(suppl 2):96–103

34. Aebli N, Krebs J, Davis G, et al. Fat embolism and acute hypotension during vertebroplasty: an experimental study in sheep. Spine 2002;27:460–466

35. Jensen ME, Evans AJ, Mathis JM, et al. Percutaneous polymethylmethacrylate vertebroplasty in the treatment of osteoporotic vertebral body compression fractures: technical aspects. AJNR Am J Neuroradiol 1997;18:1897–1904

16

Subsequent Compression Fractures after Vertebral Augmentation

JAMES S. HARROP AND ISADOR LIEBERMAN

Objectives: On completion of this chapter, the reader should be able to describe the possible reasons for remote and adjacent segment vertebral compression fractures (VCF) in elderly patients treated with vertebroplasty or kyphoplasty.

Accreditation: The American Association of Neurological Surgeons is accredited by the Accreditation Council for Continuing Medical Education to sponsor continuing medical education for physicians.

Credit: The American Association of Neurological Surgeons designates this continuing medical education activity for a maximum of 15 credits in Category I of the Physician's Recognition Award of the American Medical Association.

The Home Study Examination is online at www.aans.org/education/books/vertebro.asp

Osteoporosis is a systemic disorder characterized by bone loss and a degradation of the normal bony architecture that predisposes patients to an increased risk for fractures due to compromised bone strength. It has been further quantified, by the World Health Organization (WHO), in objective terms, as a bone density measurement less than 2.5 standard deviations below the mean value for a young adult. This disorder increases the risk of fragility fractures in ~28 million Americans. The spinal vertebrae are particularly affected by these fractures and manifest clinically as vertebral compression fractures (VCFS).

There are 1.5 million fragility fractures due to osteoporosis in the United States annually and approximately half (700,000) of these fractures affect the spine in the form of painful progressive VCFS. Compared with other spinal disorders, such as osteoarthritic back pain, this disorder is less recognized but more disabling. Only 8% of patients with osteoarthritic back problems require assistance in daily self-care, whereas over 50% of osteoporotic patients with two or more VCFs required self-care assistance.[1] Economically this disorder consumes numerous health care resources, with a projected annual cost of more than $60 billion. However, VCFs are a burden to society not only in terms of economic cost and pain, which limits activity, but also in terms of their

increased mortality rate of 24 to 34%, presumably due to respiratory compromise, compared with age-matched adults.[2,3] These statistics include correction for malignancy-related VCF. Despite these results, only one quarter to one third of patients with VCF present for medical evaluation as a result of severe pain.[2,4] Osteoporosis and compression fractures, however, are not just a major health problem of the elderly population. Secondary osteoporosis, most commonly due to iatrogenic causes, can result in similar disabilities, but typically affects a younger population. Corticosteroid medication is commonly used in the medical management of chronic obstructive pulmonary disease (COPD), autoimmune diseases, dermatologic conditions, immunosuppression after transplantation, and a multitude of other disorders. The prevalent use of steroids and their adverse affects on bone physiology results in their being the most common cause of iatrogenic secondary osteoporosis.

Approximately one third of patients who sustain a VCF have persistent pain over the region of the fracture, which is unresponsive to medical therapy. This pain can cause severe limitations in activity, resulting in significant lifestyle changes. Nonsurgical treatment options to compensate for this pain include pain medications, bracing, and bed rest. Unfortunately, in the elderly and other vulnerable fracture populations, these

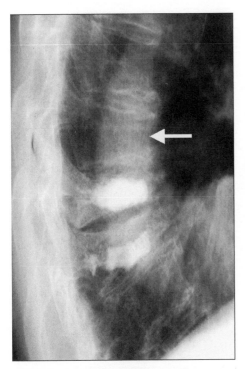

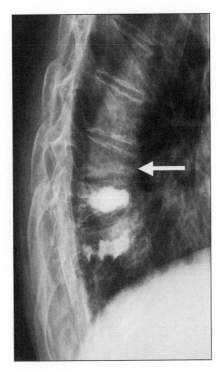

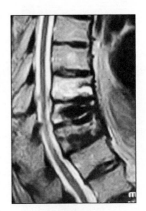

MRI 2 mo. Post-op

T8-9 Kyphoplasty   1 mo. Post-op

FIGURE 16–1 A 78-year-old woman with intractable back pain underwent a T8 and T9 kyphoplasty procedure. Postoperatively she began experiencing increasing back pain at 3 weeks. Immediate postoperative imaging shows the T8–9 kyphoplasty cement mantels in good position. Note that the T7 body has full height (arrow). Radiographs at 1 month illustrate an adjacent T7 fracture (arrow), superior to the previous kyphoplasties. Pain progressed and at 2 months' time a magnetic resonance imaging (MRI) scan (T2 sequences) shows edema in the T7 body along with further kyphosis.

strategies limit overall function and can result in significant morbidity as well as potential mortality. Vertebral augmentation with polymethylmethacrylate (PMMA) cement was originally used in the treatment of painful vertebral hemangiomas.[5] Currently, these same procedures, kyphoplasty or vertebroplasty, are being used to treat painful progressive VCFs. These techniques have been reported to improve functional outcome and significantly reduce pain scores in the short term.[6–11] Long-term results of these procedures are now being realized and are promising. Vertebroplasty involves the percutaneous injection of cement into the collapsed vertebral body. Kyphoplasty differs from vertebroplasty by first creating a cavity with an inflatable bone tamp, which indirectly restores the vertebral body height. The reduction of the kyphotic angle and spinal deformity works to restore spinal alignment, protect pulmonary function, and normalize daily function. Osteoporotic patients, after sustaining a vertebral compression fracture, have been reported to be at increased risk for a subsequent fracture.[4] A theoretical risk of vertebral augmentation is the generation of further fractures by virtue of a modulus mismatch between augmented and nonaugmented levels. The true rate of subsequent

fractures with either vertebroplasty or kyphoplasty is currently not defined.

New compression fractures, occurring after initial vertebral augmentation, can be identified based on changes from baseline imaging studies. Adjacent fractures are defined as new vertebral body compression fractures immediately rostral or caudal to a previously treated PMMA cement augmentation vertebral fracture (Fig. **16–1**). Remote fractures are defined as new compression fractures that occur with at least one vertebral body intervening between the new and the prior PMMA-treated compression fracture (Fig. **16–2**). Previously treated compression fractures are easily identified on postprocedure imaging due to the presence of the radiopaque PMMA cement in the vertebral body. Therefore, subsequent VCF cases can readily be identified on follow-up or serial radiographic evaluations.

■ Bone Loss and Biomechanics

As humans age, the ability of organ systems to compensate for changes diminishes. The skeletal system and spinal column also become more vulnerable with increased age.

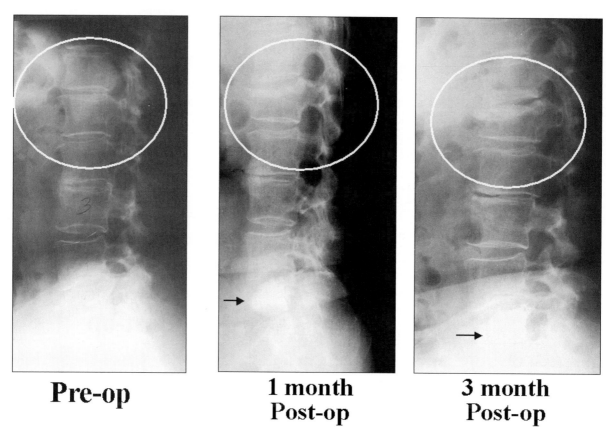

Pre-op   **1 month Post-op**   **3 month Post-op**

FIGURE 16–2 A 62-year-old man who initially presented with an L5 compression fracture. Initial plain films show the L5 compression fracture, obstructed by the iliac crest. Note that the encircled L1 vertebral body has full height. The arrow points to the successful L5 kyphoplasty. At 1 month he had increased pain at the thoracolumbar junction. Plain films show kyphotic angulation of T12 on L1 along with a superior end-plate compression fracture of L1. Three-month images showed further L1 angulation and kyphotic deformity.

There is a significant decrease in vertebral body strength resulting from the loss of cancellous bone support.[12,13] Bell et al[12] reported a direct correlation between bone loss and strength, noting that a decrease of 25% in the osseous structure resulted in a 50% decrease in vertebral strength. Rockoff and associates[14] further characterized the effects of age on loss of bone strength by analyzing the cancellous or trabecular bone's ability to compensate to applied forces. The cancellous vertebral body bone carries ~55% of axial loads in the adult spine, under the age of 40, but this percentage declines to only 35% after the age of 40.[14] These effects are manifested clinically as an ~4% annual incidence of new compression fractures in postmenopausal women (primary osteoporosis).[4] These fractures can result in a decrease in the gait velocity, an increase in muscle fatigue, and additional falls.

This degradation of bone quality on the microscopic level is compounded by the changes in the transmission of loads due to structural alterations. The thoracic and thoracolumbar regions of the spine have a natural kyphotic curvature. This curvature places the ventral thoracic spine at an increased risk for developing compression fractures as a consequence of axial loads.[15] The kyphotic curvature transmits axial forces or vectors onto the ventral portion of the vertebral body. These axial loads cause all points ventral to the vertebral body's instantaneous axis of rotation (IAR) to come closer together, while simultaneously all points dorsal to the IAR are spread apart. If the failure point of the ventral vertebral body is exceeded, a compression fracture occurs. In younger patients, significant forces are required to create a fracture, typically acquired after high-energy trauma. However, as the vertebral body is weakened by osteoporosis, the amount of energy required to initiate a fracture is significantly decreased. Once a VCF occurs, the transmission of forces through the vertebral or spinal column is altered. A VCF results in the destruction of the ventral vertebral bodies' stabilizing elements and causes the IAR to migrate dorsally to the region with intact supporting structures.[16] The dorsal migration of the IAR causes the previous mechanical advantage of a longer level arm, from which the posterior ligaments and muscles acted to maintain sagittal balance, to be shortened. The dorsal displacement of the IAR simultaneously causes the distance from the ventrally located center of gravity to the IAR to be greater, which places additional compression on the ventral columns.[16,17] Overall, the shortened dorsal lever arm working against the greater ventral bending moment arm creates a vicious cycle that places the vertebral bodies at a greater risk of further compression fractures and subsequent deformity progression.

■ Natural History of Vertebral Compression Fractures

The increased kyphotic angulation of the spine, as a result of a VCF, places the muscles and ligaments that act on the vertebral column at a biomechanical disadvantage. Clinically this is transmitted or manifested as additional compression fractures. The actual incidence of subsequent VCF following an initial fracture has been studied in postmenopausal women, who have been prospectively followed utilizing serial radiographic images. The incidence of the first compression fracture has been reported to be a rate of ~4% annually.[4] However, the greatest risk factor for a subsequent VCF is the presence of a previous VCF, because these patients have already proven that they have compromised bone structure and strength. Lindsay et al[4] retrospectively analyzed radiographs of 2725 postmenopausal women who were involved in the placebo arm of a prospective study of the effects of biphosphonate administration. Postmenopausal patients with two or more VCFs had a substantially increased risk of subsequent VCF annually. This was calculated at 19.2% when the patient had only one VCF on initial evaluation, but increased to ~24% annually as patients had two or more VCFs on their initial presentation.[4] Thus the incidence of subsequent VCF within 1 year after an index fracture in postmenopausal women rises from 4% to over 20%.

■ Postprocedural Stiffness and Fractures

Although there is little literature concerning the effect of PMMA on adjacent vertebral segments, the effects of instrumented fusions on the osteoporotic spine have been well documented. After spinal fusion there is an increased or accelerated degeneration of the vertebral bodies and disk spaces adjacent to a fusion construct.[18-22] The osteoporotic spine is particularly vulnerable after rigid spinal instrumentation, which can result in adjacent segment failure or fracture.[10]

Experimental ex vivo data have shown that PMMA augmentation increases vertebral body strength.[15,23-27] Belkoff and associates[23] further reported that the kyphoplasty balloon tamp procedures could restore the vertebral height to 97% of baseline values while concurrently restoring the vertebral body back to its initial stiffness. However, vertebral augmentation differs from fusions in that the original stiffness of the vertebral body is being restored while not altering the disk space and spinal motion characteristics. Therefore, PMMA augmentation is returning the spine to perhaps more natural biomechanical characteristics rather than fusing segments together and creating larger lever arms through which forces can act and be transmitted.

■ Vertebroplasty and Subsequent Fractures

Very little data have been accumulated about the influence of vertebroplasty and PMMA on subsequent vertebral compression fracture rates. Grados and associates[28] briefly discussed the effects of vertebroplasty on associated fractures in a small series of less than 30 patients. They reported that 52% of their patients (after following patients for a mean of 48 months) had at least one subsequent vertebral body fracture. A slight but significant increased risk of vertebral fracture in the vicinity of cemented vertebrae (odds ratio 1.44) versus fracture remote from cemented vertebrae was calculated. They postulated that this increased fracture risk was related to the change in load transfer through the spine. However, this analysis was flawed because the majority of VCFs occur in the thoracolumbar region, and in their series the treated vertebrae were clustered in the lumbar spine. Therefore, the odds ratio might be skewed by the natural selection and occurrence of the compression fractures rather than by the influence of the cemented vertebral bodies. The fractured vertebrae occurred at the transition zone from the thoracic to thoracolumbar, which is the highest area of fractures occurring, rather than the proximity to the previously augmented levels.

■ Kyphoplasty and Subsequent Fractures

As with vertebroplasty, very little data have been accumulated about the influence of kyphoplasty on subsequent VCF rates. The clinical results accumulated at our institution in the short term do not appear to increase the forces transmitted to adjacent areas despite the number of concurrent or adjacent levels treated.[29] Although vertebroplasty and kyphoplasty both strengthen the vertebral body, kyphoplasty differs in that it also aims to correct the kyphotic deformity. In principle, this should redirect the transmission of axial loads through the center of the vertebral column along the IAR. The result being a decrease in the anterior bending moment, which might lower the patient's predisposition to future compression fractures.

■ Remote and Adjacent Fractures after Kyphoplasty

At our institution, based on our experience over a 3-year period, we reviewed the influence that PMMA augmentation and deformity reduction after kyphoplasty have on the incidence of subsequent VCFs.[29] We also performed a retrospective analysis of vulnerable subpopulations of patients that had an increased incidence of subsequent fractures after kyphoplasty. Information on 115 patients' demographics, osteoporosis type, number of levels treated, follow-up period, subjective outcome scores, and office and operative reports were reviewed. All the patients'

imaging studies (pre- and postoperative) were individually reviewed and consisted of 36-inch cassettes and computed tomography (CT) and magnetic resonance imaging (MRI) scans. This information was collated into a statistical database for evaluation and statistical significance calculations.

An adjacent fracture was defined as a new fracture that occurs in the posttreatment period, either one vertebral body above or one vertebral body below the site that has been PMMA augmented (Fig. 16–1). A remote fracture was defined as any fracture to the spinal column, which was different than baseline imaging studies, that occurred a distance greater than one vertebral segment from the PMMA augmentation (Fig. 16–2). Also, a third term or "pinched" vertebral level was included in analysis and defined as a nonfractured vertebral body that was located between two treated vertebral compression fractures (Fig. 16–3). In theory, if the augmentation

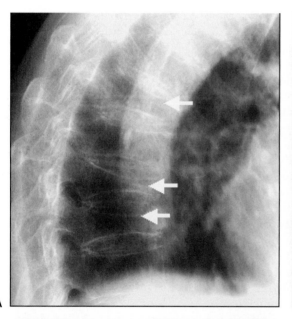

A

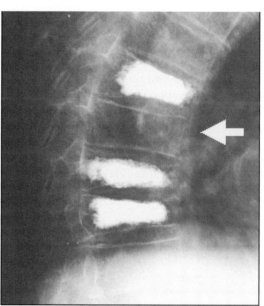

B

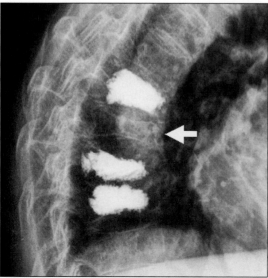

C

FIGURE 16–3 T4, T6, and T7 vertebral compression fractures **(A)**. Immediate postoperative radiograph shows T5 vertebral body with full height **(B)**. Two months postkyphoplasty an MRI T2 sequence shows a fracture in the T5 vertebral body **(C)**. This is classified as a T5 pincher (a pincher fracture).

with PMMA greatly increased the stiffness and altered spinal biomechanics, these pinched vertebral bones should have the highest incidence of subsequent fractures. Patients were followed an average of 11 months following treatment. In a range of 3 to 33 months, 25 patients developed postkyphoplasty VCFs, 18 patients had adjacent fractures, and nine patients had remote fractures. Three patients experienced both simultaneous remote and adjacent fractures. In this group the incidence of subsequent VCFs postkyphoplasty was 14.7% (33/225) per kyphoplastied vertebral body, or 21.7% per patient (25/115).

The only detailed reference on the natural history of VCF with which to compare our results was reported by Lindsay et al.[4] However, their data differ in that it was tabulated on female primary osteoporotic patients with postmenopausal VCFs. Therefore, we analyzed our patient population specifically for differences in vulnerable subpopulations. The only significant correlation was found when the patients were categorized by the etiology of their systemic osteoporosis. The primary osteoporosis population consisted of 80 patients, of whom eight patients developed postkyphoplasty fractures. This is extrapolated to an incidence of 10.8% annually (based on 11-month follow up estimated to 12 months). This population is similar to the population reflected in Lindsay et al's postmenopausal subsequent fracture data. The 10.8% postkyphoplasty subsequent fracture incidence is in fact lower than Lindsay et al's incidence of 24%. An important difference noted in the patient populations between our series and that of Lindsay et al is that the majority of patient's in our series were on concurrent medical therapy for primary osteoporosis. These agents have been shown to reduce the incidence of fractures in the osteoporotic population.[4,30] Therefore, one can determine that kyphoplasty along with concurrent medical regimens most likely maintains or lowers the subsequent incidence of adjacent fractures. There is no evidence to suggest that kyphoplasty increases the risk of subsequent fractures despite the theoretical risk of increased fractures by virtue of changing the modulus of bone.

We independently analyzed patients with secondary osteoporosis and VCFs. These patients developed osteoporosis due to treatment with chronic corticosteroids, which increase bone resorption by stimulating osteoclastogenesis.[31] There were 35 patients in this subcategory of whom 17 developed postkyphoplasty fractures (Fig. 16–4).

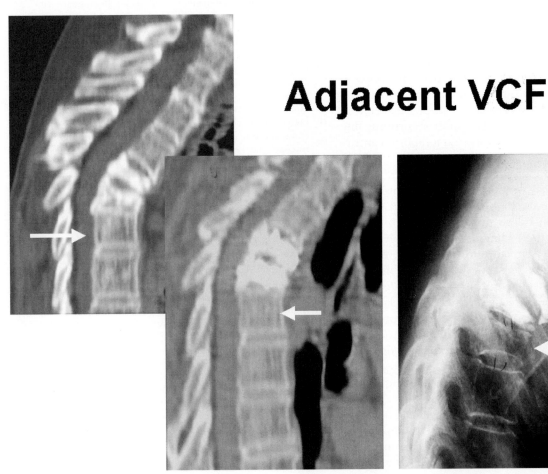

Adjacent VCF

FIGURE 16–4 A 69-year-old woman with a history of severe COPD who has been treated with chronic cortical steroid therapy. Initial films show kyphotic deformity and compression fractures at T4-T5 levels. She underwent a kyphoplasty at the T4 and T5 levels. Subsequent imaging, consisting of plain films, shows an inferior adjacent fracture of the T6 body.

This is extrapolated to a 51.2% incidence annually. Statistics were then used to further delineate differences in this subpopulation, and it was found that the corticosteroid secondary osteoporotic patients were actually younger and had a shorter follow-up period than the primary osteoporotic patients. Intuitively the younger age and shorter follow-up should bias these patients to a lower incidence of VCFs. Therefore, the high incidence of fractures noted is striking.

Osteoporotic vertebral bodies that are placed between two PMMA augmented vertebral bodies, referred to as pinched bodies (Fig. 16–3), should have the most direct forces transmitted by the increased strength from the augmented bodies. However, when analyzing the osteoporotic patients and the primary osteoporotic subgroup, it was found that these did not have a higher incidence of subsequent fractures. Interestingly the secondary or steroid-induced osteoporotic patients did have a significantly higher incidence of pinched fractures. This is most likely due to the severe weakness of the cancellous bone and the inability to repair and adapt to the increased pressure and forces applied due to the augmented vertebral bodies above or below.

■ Conclusion

The natural history of subsequent VCFs has not been fully defined, but Lindsay et al[4] retrospectively reviewed a prospective database on postmenopausal women involved in the placebo arm of osteoporosis pharmaceutical trials to address this question. This study is currently the best estimate of the natural history, and it reported an annual incidence of greater than 19.2% of subsequent VCF for patients who had more than one VCF on initial radiographs. The medical community has recognized the contribution of these fractures to morbidity and mortality, particularly in the elderly population. Vertebroplasty and kyphoplasty are two techniques that have been used to treat painful VCF refractory to medical therapy. Although these techniques to treat VCF have been shown to improve pain and outcome measures, their influence on incidence of subsequent fractures has not been clarified.

Grados et al[28] reviewed their series of vertebroplasty and reported a 52% rate of subsequent VCF. Our experience utilizing kyphoplasty and concurrent osteoporotic medical therapies has yielded a 10% rate of subsequent fractures in osteoporotic patients.[29] Interestingly, one vulnerable subpopulation has been secondary osteoporotic patients from chronic steroid therapy. These patients had a greater than 51.2% incidence of subsequent VCF.[29] The kyphoplasty protocol with concurrent medical osteoporotic regimen does not appear to increase, and in fact most likely reduces, the incidence of remote and adjacent fractures in this high-risk population. There-fore, this report argues against the theory that the further strength provided through methylmethacrylate augmentation results in an increased degradation of the other vertebral bodies—at least in the short-term.

REFERENCES

1. Leidig-Bruckner G, Minne HW, Schlaich C, et al. Clinical grading of spinal osteoporosis: quality of life components and spinal deformity in women with chronic low back pain and women with vertebral osteoporosis. J Bone Miner Res 1997;12:663–675
2. Cooper C. The crippling consequences of fractures and their impact on quality of life. Am J Med 1997;103:12S–17S
3. Kado DM, Bowner WS, Palermo L, Nevitt MC, Genant HK, Cummings SR. Vertebral fractures and mortality in older women: a prospective study. Arch Intern Med 1999;159:1215–1220
4. Lindsay R, Silverman SL, Cooper C, et al. Risk of new vertebral fracture in the year following a fracture. JAMA 2001;285: 320–323
5. Galibert P, Deramond H, Rosat P, Le Gars D. [Preliminary note on the treatment of vertebral angioma by percutaneous acrylic vertebroplasty] (in French). Neurochirurgie 1987;33:166–168
6. Barr JD, Barr MS, Lemley TJ, McCann RM. Percutaneous vertebroplasty for pain relief and spinal stabilization. Spine 2000;25: 923–928
7. Cyteval C, Sarrabere MP, Roux JO, et al. Acute osteoporotic vertebral collapse: open study on percutaneous injection of acrylic surgical cement in 20 patients. AJR Am J Roentgenol 1999;173: 1685–1690
8. Garfin SR, Yuan HA, Reiley MA. New technologies in spine: kyphoplasty and vertebroplasty for the treatment of painful osteoporotic compression fractures. Spine 2001;26:1511–1515
9. Jensen ME, Evans AJ, Mathias J, Kallmes DF, Cloft HJ, Dion JE. Percutaneous polymethyl-methacrylate vertebroplasty in the treatment of osteoporotic vertebral body compression fractures: technical aspects. AJNR Am J Neuroradiol 1997;18:1897–1904
10. Lieberman IH, Dudeney S, Reinhardt MK, Bell G. Initial outcome and efficacy of "kyphoplasty" in the treatment of painful osteoporotic vertebral compression fractures. Spine 2001;26: 1631–1638
11. Wong W, Reiley MA, Garfin S. Vertebroplasty/kyphoplasty. J Women's Health 2000;2:117–124
12. Bell GH, Dunbar O, Beck JS, Gibb A. Variations in strength of vertebrae with age and their relation to osteoporosis. Calcif Tissue Res 1967;1:75–86
13. Perry O. Fracture of the vertebral end-plate in the lumbar spine. Acta Orthop Scand 1957;25:34–39
14. Rockoff SD, Sweet E, Bleustein J. The relative contribution of trabecular and cortical bone to the strength of human lumbar vertebrae. Calcif Tissue Res 1969;3:163–175
15. Heini PF, Walchli B, Berlemann U. Percutaneous transpedicular vertebroplasty with PMMA: operative technique and early results: a prospective study for the treatment of osteoporotic compression fractures. Eur Spine J 2000;9:445–450
16. Haher TR, Bergman M, O'Brien M, et al. The effect of the three columns of the spine on the instantaneous axis of rotation in flexion and extension. Spine 1991;16(8 suppl):S312–S318
17. Haher TR, O'Brien M, Felmly WT, et al. Instantaneous axis of rotation as a function of the three columns of the spine. Spine 1992;17(6 suppl):S149–S154
18. Hilibrand AS, Yoo JU, Carlson GD, et al. The success of anterior cervical arthrodesis adjacent to a previous fusion. Spine 1997; 22:1574–1579
19. Hunter LY, Braunstein EM, Bailey RR. Radiographic changes following anterior cervical fusion. Spine 1980;5:399–401

20. Etebar S, Cahill DW. Risk factors for adjacent-segment failure following lumbar fixation with rigid instrumentation for degenerative instability. J Neurosurg Spine 1999;90:163–169

21. Perez-Grueso FS, Fernandez-Baillo N, de Robles SA, Fernandez AG, Bridwell KH, DeWald RL. The low lumbar spine below Cotrel-Dubousset instrumentation long–term findings. Spine 2000;25: 2333–2341

22. Takahashi S, Delecrin J, Passuti N. Changes in the unfused lumbar spine in patients with idiopathic scoliosis. A 5- to 9-year assessment after Cotrel-Dubousset instrumentation. Spine 1997;22:517–523; discussion: 524

23. Belkoff SM, Mathis JM, Fenton DC, et al. An ex vivo biomechanical evaluation of an inflatable bone tamp used in the treatment of compression fractures Spine 2001;26:151–156

24. Belkoff SM, Mathis JM, Jasper LE, Deramond H. An ex vivo biomechanical evaluation of a hydroxyapatite cement for use with vertebroplasty. Spine 2001;26:1542–1546

25. Dean JR, Ison KT, Gishen P. The strengthening effect of percutaneous vertebroplasty. Clin Radiol 2000;55:471–476

26. Liebschner MA, Rosenberg WS, Keaveny TM. Effects of bone cement volume and distribution on vertebral stiffness after vertebroplasty. Spine 2001;26:1547–1554

27. Tohmeh AG, Mathis JM, Fenton DC, Levine AM, Belkoff SM. Biomechanical efficacy of unipedicular versus bipedicular vertebroplasty for the management of osteoporotic compression fractures. Spine 1999;24:1772–1776

28. Grados F, Depriester C, Cayrolle G, Hardy N, Deramond H, Fardellone P. Long-term observations of vertebral osteoporotic fractures treated by percutaneous vertebroplasty. Rheumatology (Oxf) 2000;39:1410–1414

29. Harrop JS, Lieberman I, Reinhart MK, Prpa B. Steroid induced secondary osteoporosis relationship to subsequent compression fractures after kyphoplasty. Eur Spine J 2002;11:S22

30. Dunn CJ, Fitton A, Sorkin EM. Etidronic acid. A review of its pharmacological properties and therapeutic efficacy in the resorptive bone disease. Drugs Aging 1994;5:446–474

31. Canalis E, Delany AM. Mechanisms of glucocorticoid action in bone. Ann N Y Acad Sci 2002;966:73–81

Index